WHERE THERE S
A WILL
THERE IS
A WAFFLE

20 low carb and gluten free
waffle recipes for a ketogenic diet.

By: Paul Spalding

ISBN 13 - 978-1-7323210-0-7

Photography by: Paul Spalding
Cover design by: Paul Spalding
Recipes by: Paul Spalding
Everything by: Paul Spalding

Printed in United States of America

For more info or to contact the author, visit ShreddedRedwood.com

Dedicated to the memory of:

Michael "Smaaaaaaaaaaaaa" Smith

Thanks for showing me how to go after a dream, no matter the odds.

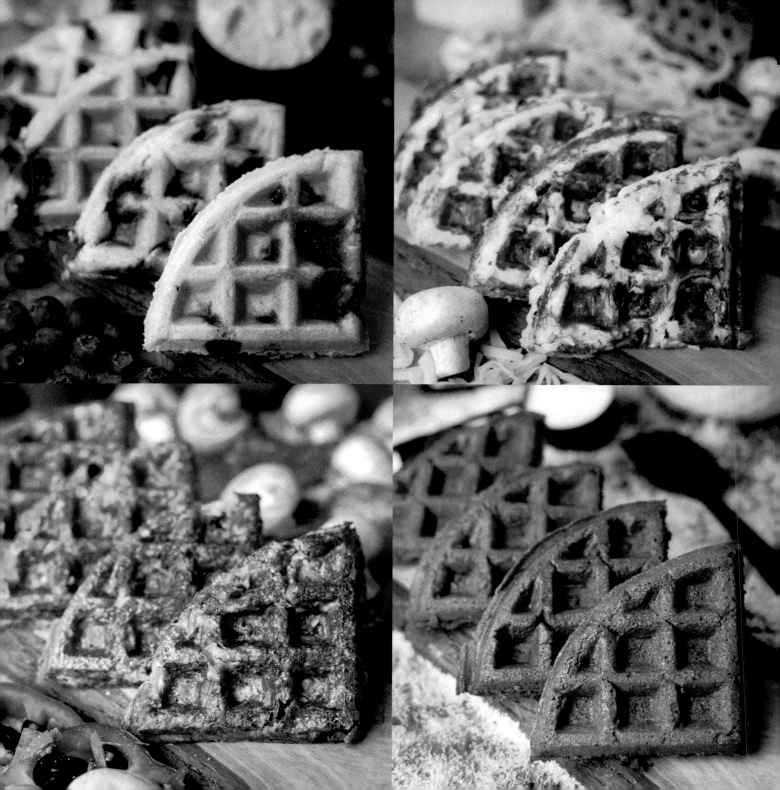

Table Of Contents

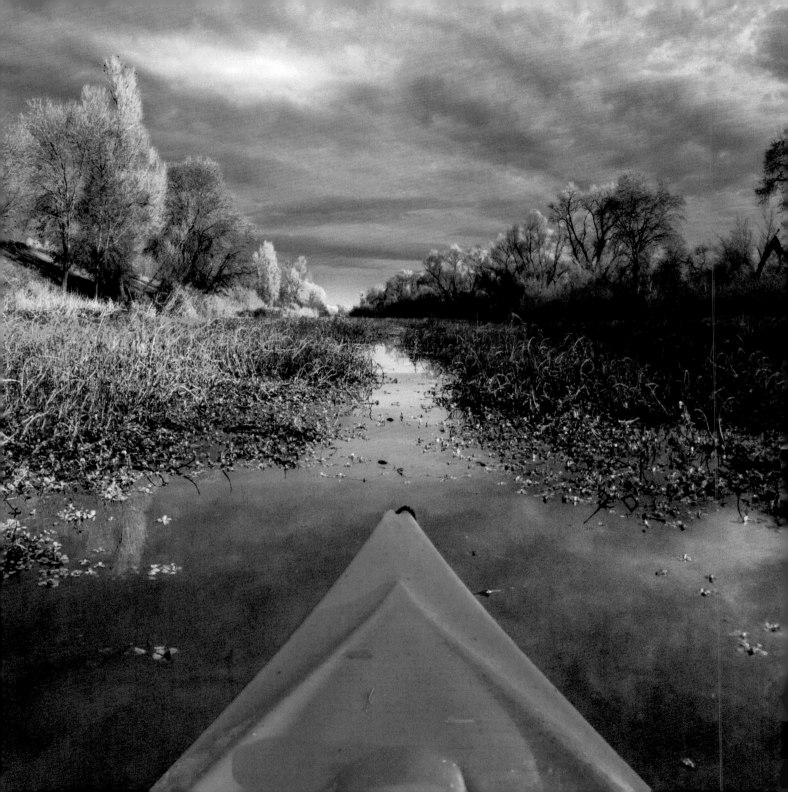

Why Waffles?

After spending years on a Ketogenic diet, I was always trying to track down foods with a quality crunch to them. While working on a cauliflower pizza recipe one day, I couldn't quite get that classic crisp that I was looking for. So I tossed a slice in a frying pan to give it more crunch. The realization of the cheese from the "crust" crisping up from the hot frying pan had me wondering if I could do that with the entire pizza. Then came the waffle iron. It was the perfect utensil for my goals. A hot surface to heat, fry and crisp all the areas of my pizza plans! I threw some things in a bowl, waffled it up and the first pepperoni pizza waffle was born. Little did I know that first experiment and journey down wacky waffle iron lane would result in months and months of waffles for every meal. I know what you're thinking, "He can't really mean every meal.". Every. Meal. It was definitely a journey of ups and downs with plenty of pretty bad waffles. Luckily, this book is a culmination of all the greats and none of the flops. All the waffles that made my body, brain and taste buds go, "Mmm, that's niiiice.". There's not many foods that I miss on a low carb diet, but this book was written to fill the void with a hot sizzle and a tasty crunch. To prove that even during a time of wanting a cheat, if there's a will to succeed, there is a waffle.

About the Author

Paul Spalding is a personal trainer, photographer, outdoor adventurer, lover of creative cooking and a ketogenic diet. Having spent most of his youth slamming back gas station soda buckets and corn dogs, he grew up thinking he was destined to always be, "the big guy". In 2012, at the age of twenty-four he decided to change that mindset. With three years of experience in a small restaurant and an overall love for getting risky in the kitchen, he buckled down. One year, and seventy pounds later his goal was reached and life changed. Now he's a personal trainer and advocate for people getting outdoors and getting in shape. He still follows a ketogenic diet while trail running, kayaking and mountain biking for the perfect nature photo. His photography, training services and other recipes can be found at ShreddedRedwood.com.

Special thanks to my friends and brother for putting up with me sending them drool inducing waffle photos all the time, my dog and roommate for helping me taste test and my awesome Mom for encouraging to stand out from the rest, in life and in the process of writing this book. Y'all are awesome and I wouldn't be who I am without you around.

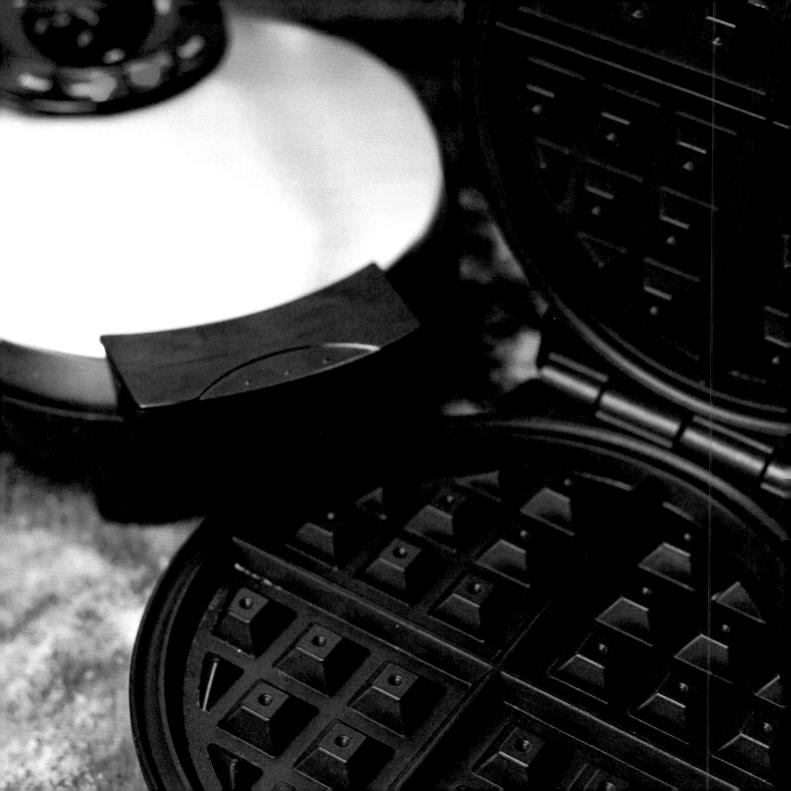

Explaining The Iron

I wrote this book while using an 8-inch Belgian waffle iron with an adjustable temperature. Different irons sizes might yield different outcomes in waffle size and cook time but the flavors and crunch will still be the same. Some recipes require temperatures other than 100%, if your iron doesn't have that ability to be adjusted, a few of the recipes won't be achievable.

Waffle Words

Waffle Wells:

The deepest depths of the waffle iron. From between the dimples to the edge of the iron.

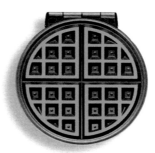

Waffle Ridges:

The section that runs along the inner edges of each individual waffle triangle.

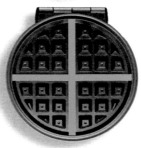

Removing Your Waffles

Individually

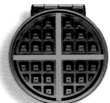

Use a rubber spatula to cut the waffle along the waffle ridges. Remove one at a time by lifting the waffle along the outer waffle wells, sliding a spatula under and lifting each one individually to a cutting board or cooling rack.

As a Whole

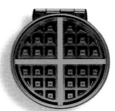

Remove by lifting an edge with a fork at the tip of a waffle ridge. Slide a spatula underneath and towards the center. Lift / slide to a cutting board or cooling rack.

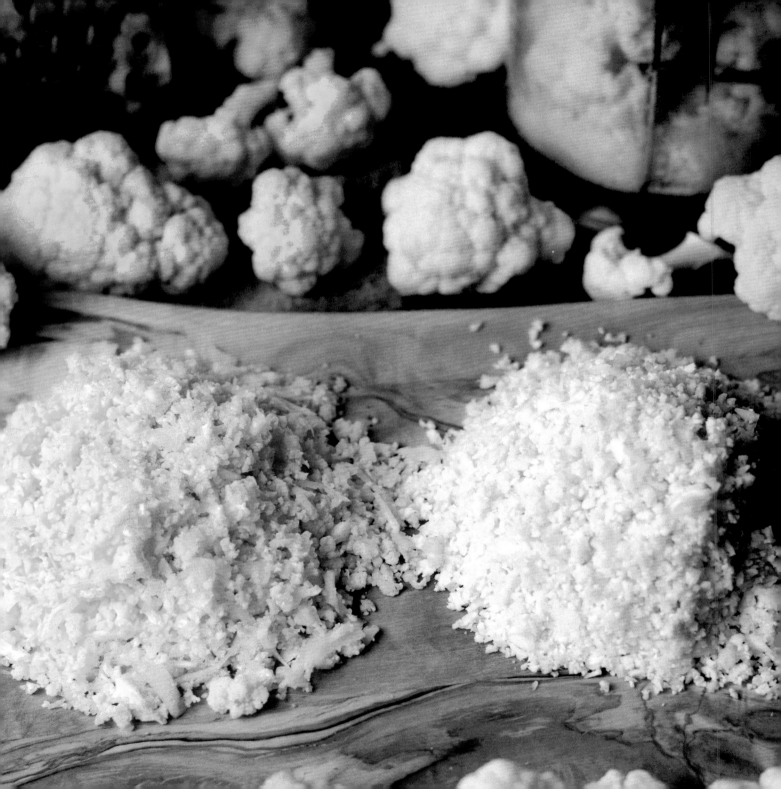

Making Riced Cauliflower

Since this book has several recipes that call for different measurements of riced cauliflower, I decided I should probably dedicate a page to the simplicity of making your own riced cauliflower. It can be done for relatively cheap, is a great way to add nutrients to a recipe and, well, you're going to need it for quite a few recipes in this book.

A medium sized head should make around 6 cups of riced cauliflower.

Cheese Grater

This process will make slightly larger chunks of riced cauliflower and take a little more work, it's still a good way of making what's needed for these recipes. Remove the excess vegetation (leaves, extra stem, etc.). Break it down into the individual florets. Toss into a strainer and rinse under water. Run the florets down the larger grates of the cheese grater as if you're grating cheese. Careful to be mindful of hands and knuckles while doing so, you'll want to start with the top of the floret and work your way towards the inner part of the stem.

Food Processor

The easiest way to make your riced cauliflower (other than buying premade). Remove the excess vegetation (leaves, extra stem, etc.). Break it down into the individual florets. Toss into a strainer and rinse under water. Slice into smaller pieces, place into a blender or food processor and pulse till riced. Sometimes larger pieces can get stuck to the walls so it may be useful to check after a pulse or two. Use a rubber spatula to move the larger pieces around for better blending. You'll want to aim for turning it into a fine rice like consistency so a couple pulses should do, but your processor and floret size may vary.

Storage

Riced Cauliflower can be stored in tupperware or ziplock bags in the fridge for 4-5 days or up to 6 months in the freezer.

Measuring

Using the riced cauliflower in its raw form means it's going to have a higher moisture content. When measuring, it should be "packed" into the measuring cup or spoon and then leveled off the top with a knife or other flat surface. Similar to if you were measuring brown sugar.

Pre-riced frozen cauliflower?

Since the prepacked frozen riced cauliflower is flash frozen, it has too much moisture to it for these recipes. Even if you were to let it thaw before hand, you'd still end up with one soggy waffle. Though, some stores do carry pre-riced that hasn't been flash frozen, so keep an eye out if you'd like the easy route.

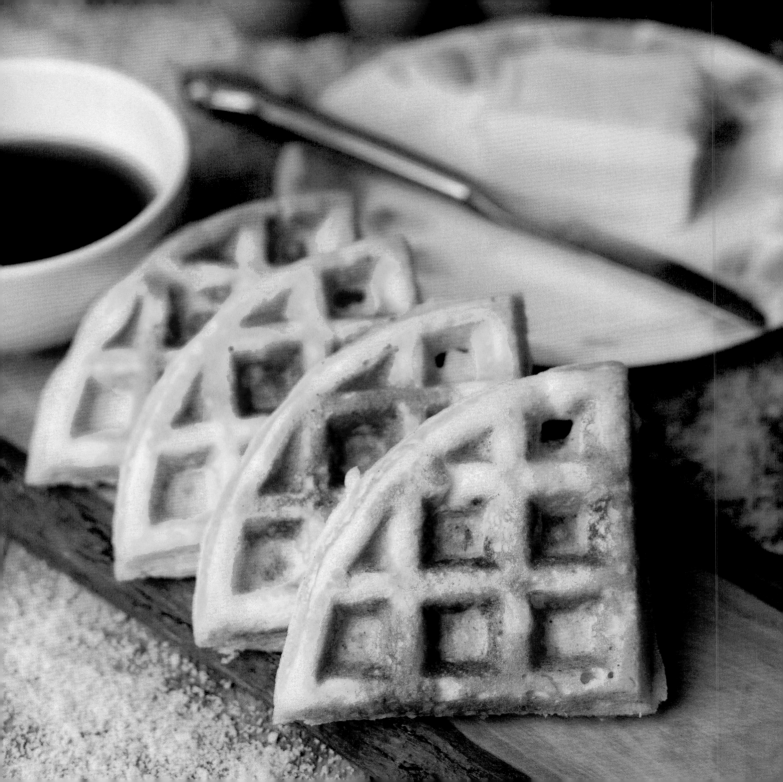

ALMOND FLOUR CLASSIC

What would a book of waffles be without a classic? Simple, buttery, light and crispy. The almond flour classic is basic waffle without all the gluten and carbs. Enjoy with some syrup or use it as the outer "bread" for your favorite breakfast sandwich.

Prep: 5 Minutes	Cook: 1.5 - 2 Minutes	Total: 7 Minutes

Almond Flour	2/3 Cup
Salt	1/4 Tsp
Baking Powder	1/4 Tsp
Heavy Whipping Cream	3 Tbsp
Melted Butter	2 Tbsp
Large Egg(s)	1

Plug in a clean waffle iron and set the temperature to **100% heat.**

In a medium sized mixing bowl, stir together the almond flour, salt and baking powder.

In the same mixing bowl, stir in the heavy whipping cream, melted butter and egg

Using a rubber spatula, pour the waffle batter into the center of the iron.

Spread the ingredients to the edges of the waffle wells and close the iron. **Bake briefly for 1½ - 2 minutes on 100% heat.**

Lift the lid to check for desired color. Remove by lifting an edge with a fork at the tip of a waffle ridge. Slide a spatula underneath and towards the center. Lift / slide to a cutting board or cooling rack.

Allow to cool briefly and enjoy!

Tips: **Freeze Them!** Store any leftovers in the freezer! Re-heat in an iron or toaster oven!

Make it meaty: Add 2 Tbsp of crumbled bacon to the top of the batter before closing the lid.

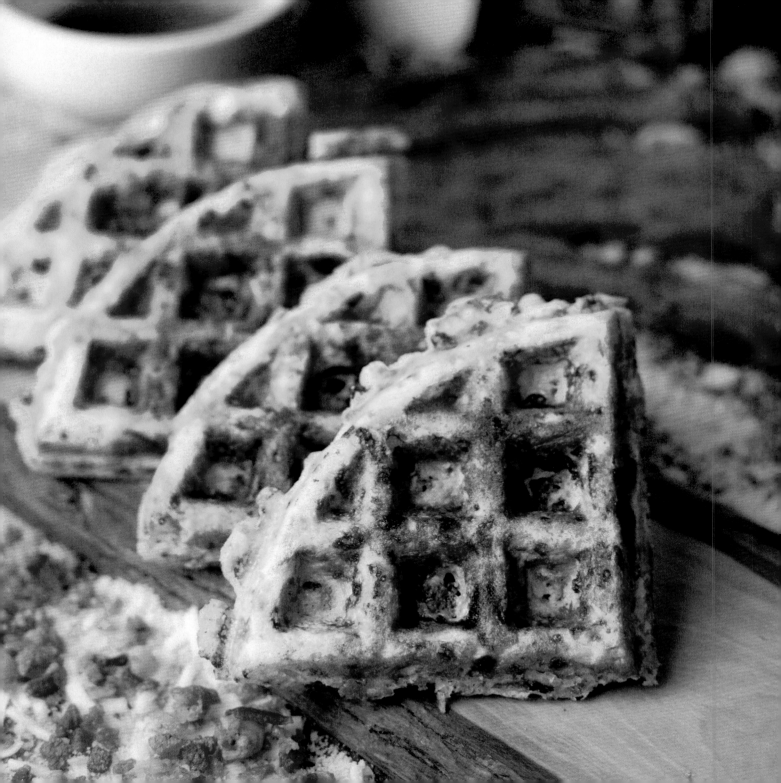

MAPLE BACON

No more need to use both hands for your bacon and waffles while simultaneously trying to figure out how you're going to get syrup into the equation. The Maple Bacon Waffle brings all those worlds into one delicious, hand held and crunchy waffle for the bacon loving multitasker.

Prep: 5 Minutes	Cook: 5 Minutes	Total: 10 Minutes

Almond Flour	1/2 Cup
Shredded Mozzarella Cheese	1/2 Cup
Crumbled Bacon	1/4 Cup
Salt	1/4 Tsp
Sugar Free Maple Syrup	2 Tbsp
Heavy Whipping Cream	2 Tbsp
Large Egg(s)	1

Plug in a clean waffle iron and set the temperature to **100% heat.**

In a medium sized mixing bowl, stir together the almond flour, cheese, crumbled bacon and salt.

In the same mixing bowl, stir in the sugar free maple syrup, heavy whipping cream and egg.

Using a rubber spatula, pour / scoop the waffle batter into the center of the iron.

Spread the ingredients to the edges of the waffle wells and close the iron with a light press to the top to make sure all ingredients are spread evenly. Be careful not to press the hot parts of the iron. **Bake for around 5 minutes on 100% heat.**

Lift the lid to check for desired color. Remove by lifting an edge with a fork at the tip of a waffle ridge. Slide a spatula underneath and towards the center. Lift / slide to a cutting board or cooling rack.

Allow to cool briefly and enjoy!

Tips: **Don't feel like cooking bacon?** Real bacon bits will totally work too!

Make it meaty-er: Mix it up with 2 Tbsp cooked sausage and 2 Tbsp crumbled bacon instead.

MAPLE BACON
BACON & EGG SANDWICH

Cook some bacon.
Fry an egg.
Stack between two Maple Bacon waffles (hot or cold).
You've got yourself a Breakfast sandwich.

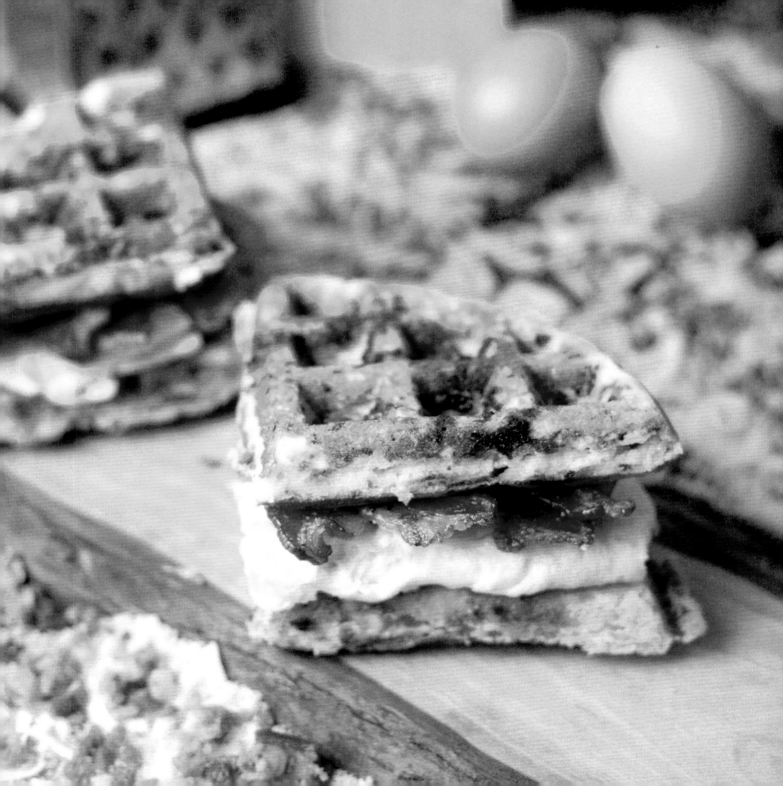

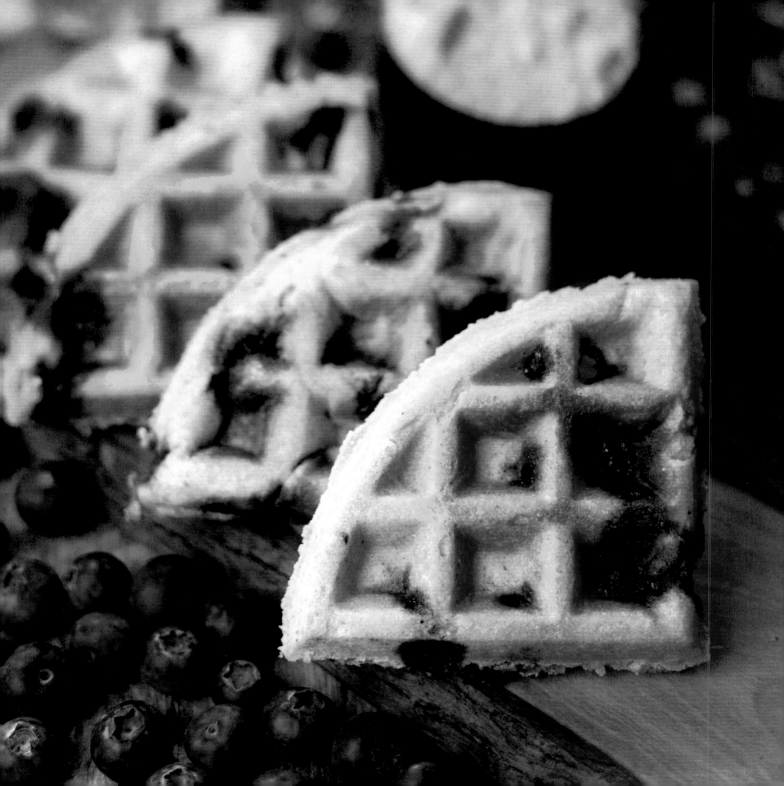

BLUEBERRY MUFFIN

I honestly thought this waffle was gonna to drive me crazy. I made so many variations before I was finally able nail the perfect crumbly, yet moist muffin texture. From too dry to a bit too cakey, I waffled them all before pinpointing this perfect combination of buttery blueberry goodness that falls apart in your mouth.

Prep: 5 Minutes	Cook: 15 Minutes	Total: 25 Minutes

Almond Flour	1/2 Cup
Coconut Flour	2 Tbsp
Pyure Stevia Blend	3 Tbsp
Melted Butter	4 Tbsp
Large Egg Whites(s)	3
Frozen Blueberries	1/2 Cup

Plug in a clean waffle iron and set the temperature to **25% heat.**

In a medium sized mixing bowl, stir together the almond flour, coconut flour and stevia.

In the same mixing bowl, stir in the melted butter and egg whites.

Mix the frozen blueberries into the batter. This will likely cause the batter to thicken up quite considerably and allow the dough to be shaped into more of a ball.

Using a rubber spatula, roll the waffle dough from the bowl into the center of the iron. Lightly moisten your fingers to prevent sticking and press the waffle dough evenly to the edges of the waffle wells.

Close your iron with a light press to the top to make sure all ingredients are spread evenly. Be careful not to press the hot parts of the iron. **Bake for around 15 minutes on 25% heat.**

Lift the lid to check for a golden brown or a bit darker. Unplug the waffle iron.

Allow the waffle iron to cool for around 5 minutes. Using a rubber spatula, cut the waffle along the ridges. Remove one at a time by lifting the waffle along the outer waffle wells, sliding a spatula under and lifting each one individually to a cutting board or cooling rack.

Enjoy!

Tips: **Make it raspberry:** Swap out the blueberries for a 1/2 Cup of frozen raspberries.

No coconut? Use an extra 2 Tbsp almond flour. It'll be a little less muffin like, but still great!

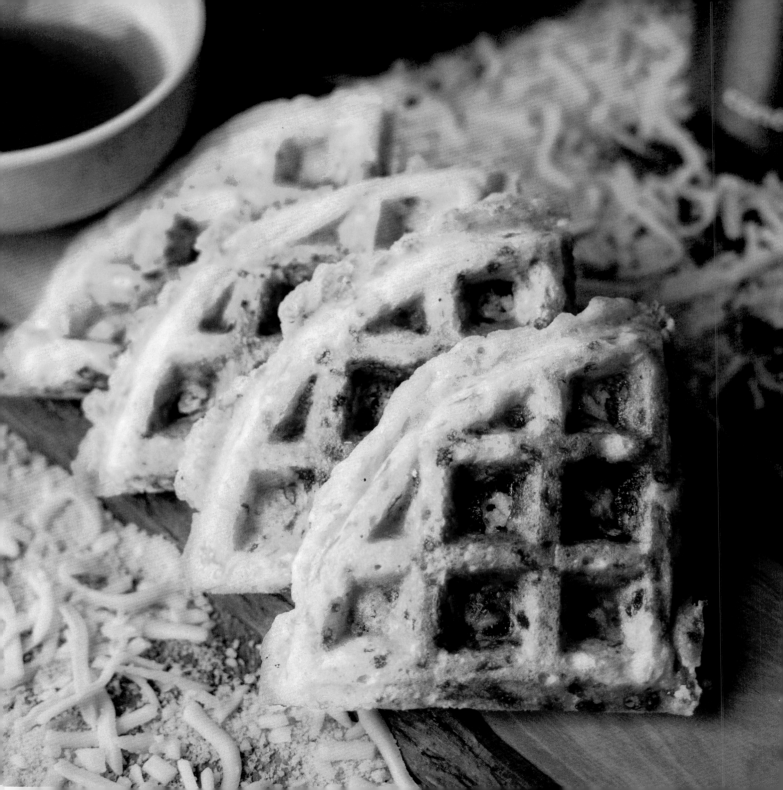

MAPLE ON-THE-GO

From the first moment this batter sizzles into the wells of the iron to the final bite, that familiar maple flavor fills your senses. Creamy, crunchy, gooey and sweet all at the same time, the maple on the go is a breakfast classic anywhere you need it to be.

Prep: 5 Minutes	Cook: 4 Minutes	Total: 9 Minutes

Almond Flour	1/2 Cup
Shredded Mozzarella Cheese	3/4 Cup
Salt	1/4 Tsp
Sugar Free Maple Syrup	4 Tbsp
Large Egg(s)	1

Plug in a clean waffle iron and set the temperature to **50% heat.**

In a medium sized mixing bowl, stir together the almond flour, cheese and salt.

In the same mixing bowl, stir in the sugar free maple syrup and egg.

Using a rubber spatula, pour the waffle batter into the center of the iron.

Spread the ingredients to the edges of the waffle wells and close the iron with a light press to the top to make sure all ingredients are spread evenly. Be careful not to touch the hot parts of the iron. **Bake for around 4 minutes on 50% heat.**

Lift the lid to check for desired color. Remove by lifting an edge with a fork at the tip of a waffle ridge. Slide a spatula underneath and towards the center. Lift / slide to a cutting board or cooling rack.

Allow to cool briefly and enjoy!

Tips: **Freeze Them!** Store any leftovers in the freezer! Re-heat in an iron or toaster oven!

Looking for a little bit more crunch? Let it cook a bit longer.

MAPLE ON-THE-GO
SAUSAGE & EGG
BREAKFAST SANDWICH

Cook a sausage patty.
fry an egg.
Stack between two Maple On-The-Go waffles (hot or cold).
You've got yourself a sandwich.

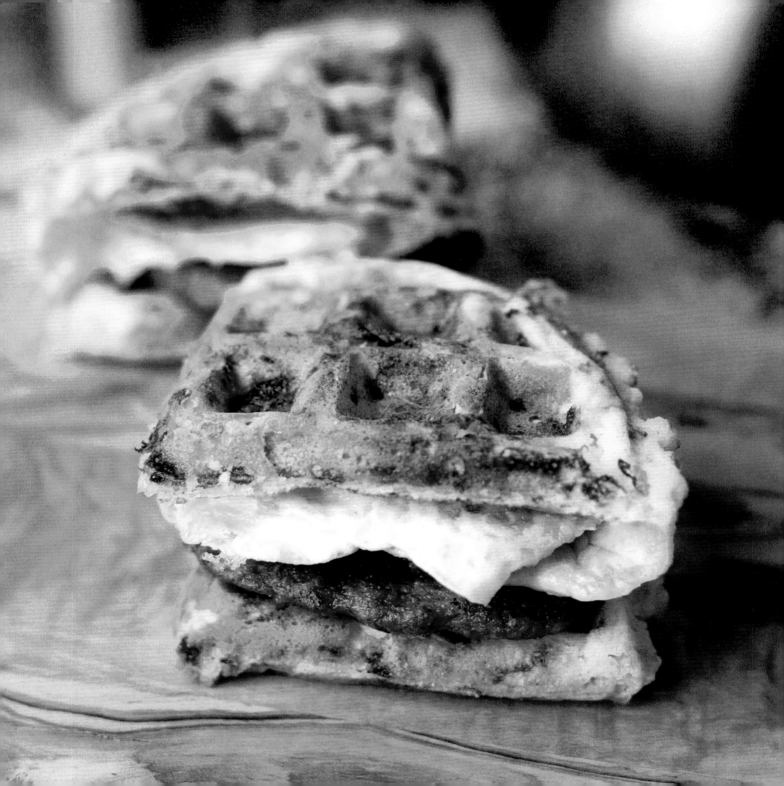

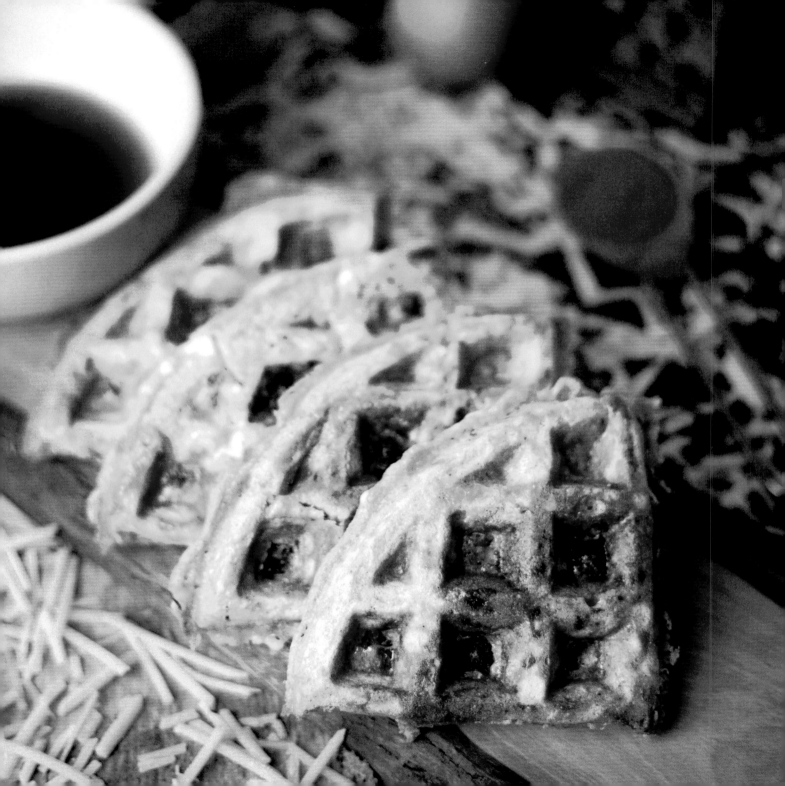

FRENCH TOAST

Going low carb use to mean missing out on the amazing flavor and texture of a good French toast. Well, not anymore! The cottage cheese adds a familiar eggy bread like texture while the hot waffle iron steams out the amazingly familiar cinnamon smell.

Prep: 5 Minutes	Cook: 4 Minutes	Total: 9 Minutes

Almond Flour	1/3 Cup
Shredded Mozzarella Cheese	1/4 Cup
Shredded Parmesan Cheese	1/4 Cup
Stevia	1 1/2 Tsp
Cinnamon	3/4 Tsp
Sugar Free Maple Syrup	2 Tbsp
Cottage Cheese	2 Tbsp
Large Egg(s)	1

Plug in a clean waffle iron and set the temperature to **75% heat.**

In a medium sized mixing bowl, mix together the almond flour, cheese, stevia and cinnamon.

In the same mixing bowl, mix in the sugar free maple syrup, cottage cheese and egg.

Using a rubber spatula, pour / scoop the waffle batter into the center of the iron and spread the ingredients to the edges of the waffle wells. This recipe has a tendency to stick to the top of the iron. For best results use a nonstick spray or lightly grease the top of the iron before closing the lid.

Close the waffle iron with a slight press to make sure it's all evenly spread out. Be careful not to press the hot parts of the iron. **Bake for around 4 minutes on 75% heat.**

Open the iron slow and steady to allow the weight of the waffle to keep things from sticking or pulling apart and unplug the waffle iron.

Allow the iron to cool for around 5 minutes. Use a rubber spatula to cut the waffle into individual triangles along the waffle ridges. Remove one at a time by lifting the waffle along the outer waffle wells, sliding a spatula under and lifting each one individually to a cutting board or cooling rack.

 Tips: **Do I really need to grease the iron to make sure it doesn't stick?** yes.

Let it cool! This is one of the waffles that takes on a different texture as it cools down.

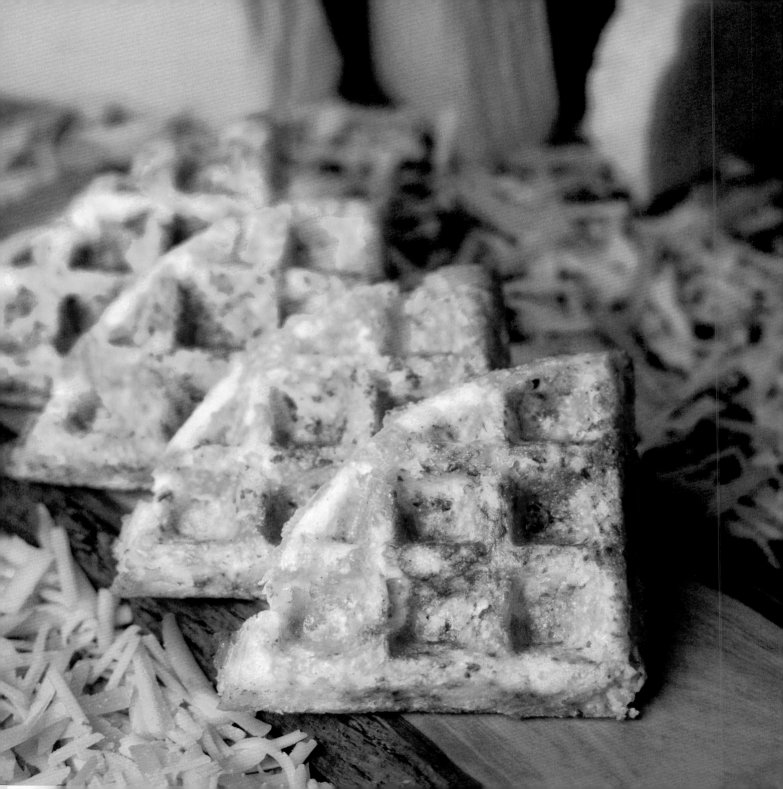

THREE CHEESE

Cheese, who doesn't love cheese? Nothing like cherishing cheesy cheddar goodness mixed into a molten mozzarella melt that's permeating a parmesan perfection of flavor. Three cheeses, one waffle, a whole lot of goodness.

Prep: 5 Minutes	Cook: 4 Minutes	Total: 9 Minutes

Almond Flour	3 Tbsp
Raw Riced Cauliflower	1/2 Cup
Shredded Mozzarella Cheese	1/4 Cup
Shredded Mild Cheddar Cheese	1/4 Cup
Shredded Parmesan Cheese	1/4 Cup
Salt	1/4 Tsp
Large Egg(s)	1

Plug in a clean waffle iron and set the temperature to **100% heat.**

- -

In a medium sized mixing bowl, stir together the almond flour, raw riced cauliflower, cheese and salt.

- -

In the same mixing bowl, stir in the egg.

Using a rubber spatula, pour / scoop the waffle batter into the center of the iron. Lightly moisten your fingers to prevent sticking and press the waffle dough evenly to the edges of the waffle wells.

- -

Close the iron with a light press to the top to make sure all ingredients are spread evenly. Be careful not to press the hot parts of the iron. **Bake briefly for around 4 minutes on 100% heat.**

- -

Lift the lid to check for desired color. Remove by lifting an edge with a fork at the tip of a waffle ridge. Slide a spatula underneath and towards the center. Lift / slide to a cutting board or cooling rack.

- -

Allow to cool briefly and enjoy!

 Tips:

Make it pesto: Add 1 Tbsp pesto sauce for an added twist.

Change up the Cheeses: Try swapping out the mozzarella for pepperjack for some spice.

THREE CHEESE
GRILLED CHEESE

Grate some cheese.
Set your waffle iron to 25% heat.
Place half of a Three Cheese Waffle in the front half of your iron.
Place grated cheese on top of the waffles.
Stack the other half of waffle on top.
Close your iron lightly and allow to cook till the cheese is melted.
You've got yourself a sandwich.

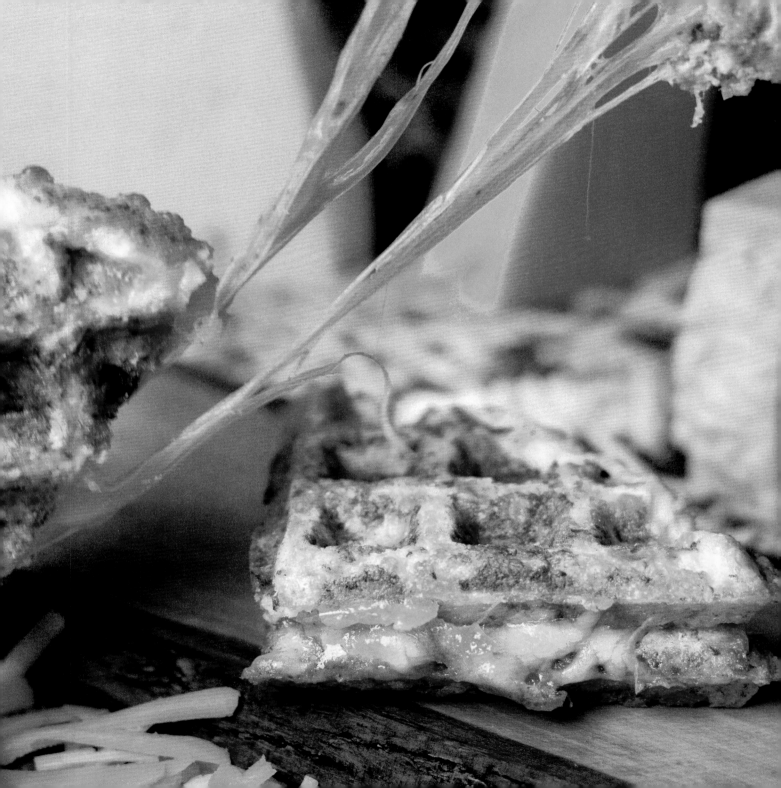

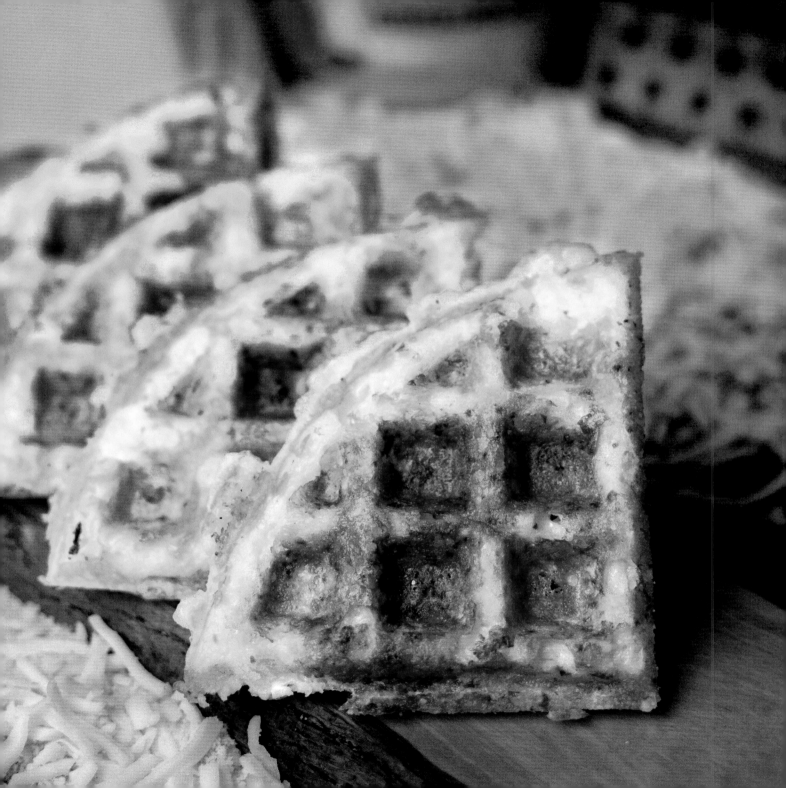

PEPPER JACK RANCH

The perfect way to achieve the crunch, slight spice and contrasting cooling effect of a pepper jack grilled cheese sandwich with a side of ranch, without all the carbs or mess.

Prep: 5 Minutes	Cook: 4 Minutes	Total: 9 Minutes

Almond Flour	1/4 Cup
Riced Cauliflower	1/4 Cup
Shredded Parmesan Cheese	1/4 Cup
Shredded Pepper jack Cheese	1/2 Cup
Salt	1/4 Tsp
Ranch	2 Tbps
Large Egg(s)	1

Plug in a clean waffle iron and set the temperature to **100% heat.**

In a medium sized mixing bowl, stir together the almond flour, raw riced cauliflower, cheese and salt.

In the same mixing bowl, stir in the ranch dressing and egg.

Using a rubber spatula, pour / scoop the waffle batter into the center of the iron. Lightly moisten your fingers to prevent sticking and press the waffle dough evenly to the edges of the waffle wells.

Close the iron with a light press to the top to make sure all ingredients are spread evenly. Be careful not to press the hot parts of the iron. **Bake briefly for around 4 minutes on 100% heat.**

Lift the lid to check for desired color. Remove by lifting an edge with a fork at the tip of a waffle ridge. Slide a spatula underneath and towards the center. Lift / slide to a cutting board or cooling rack.

Allow to cool briefly and enjoy!

Tips: **Freeze Them!** Store any leftovers in the freezer! Re-heat in an iron or toaster oven!

Looking for more spice? Add 1 Tbsp canned and drained diced green chillies or jalapenos.

PEPPER JACK RANCH
BACON LETTUCE TOMATO

Cook some bacon.
Slice up a tomato.
Tear off some lettuce.
Stack between two Pepper Jack Ranch waffles (hot or cold).
No mayo needed.
You've got yourself a sandwich.

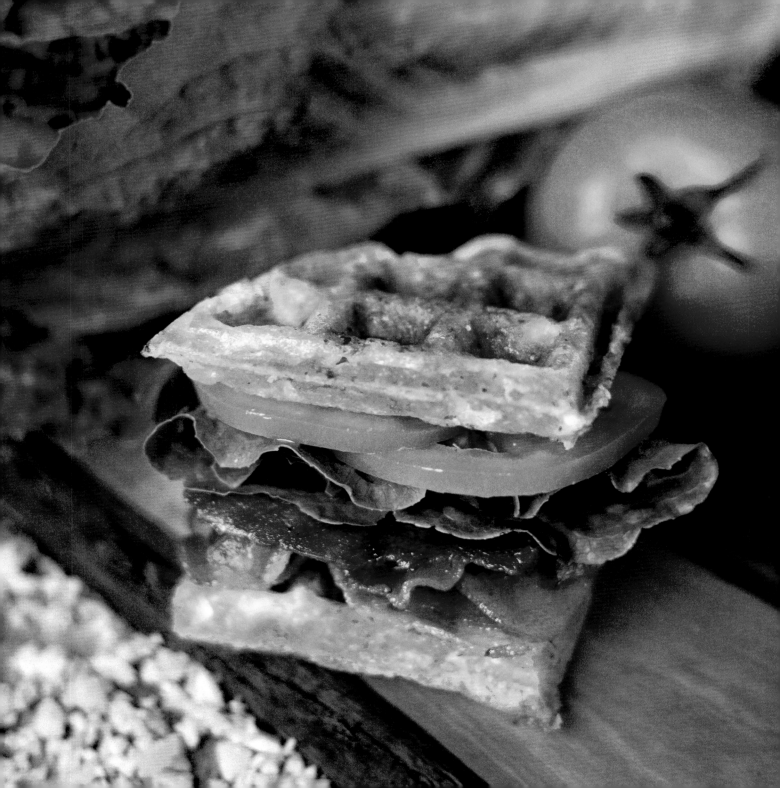

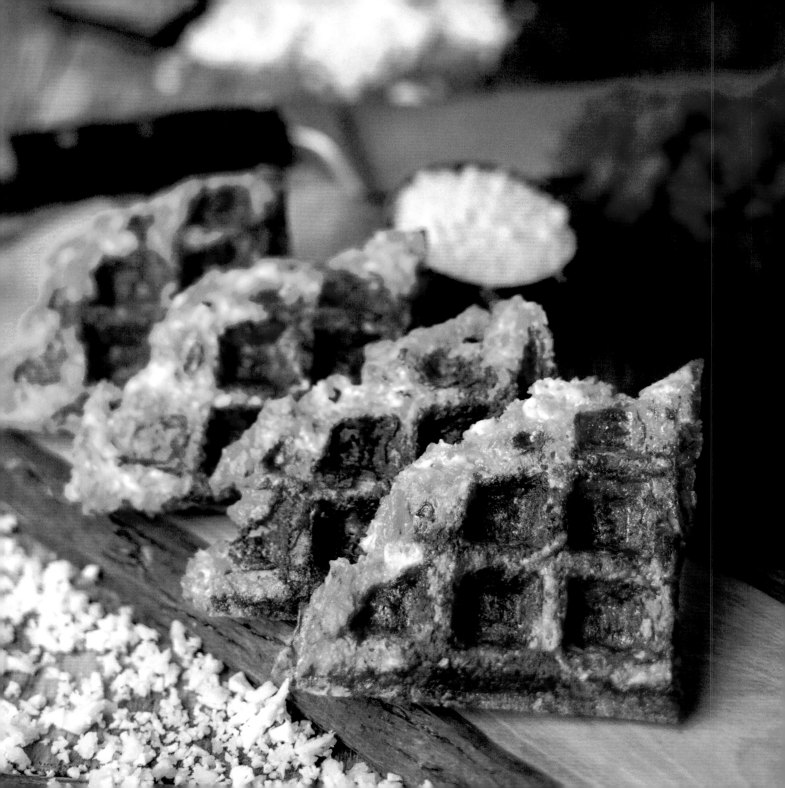

PEPPERONI PIZZA

The Waffle that started it all! No more soggie excuses for pizza!
The pepperoni pizza waffle brings back the tasty pepperoni crunch without the carbs.

Prep: 5 Minutes	Cook: 3 Minutes	Total: 8 Minutes

Almond Flour	1/4 Cup
Raw Riced Cauliflower	1/4 Cup
Shredded Parmesan Cheese	1/4 Cup
Shredded Pepper Jack Cheese	1/2 Cup
Minced Pepperoni	1/4 Cup
Salt	1/4 Tsp
Tomato Paste	2 Tbsp
Large Egg(s)	1

Plug in a clean waffle iron and set the temperature to **100% heat.**

In a medium sized mixing bowl, stir together the almond flour, raw riced cauliflower, cheese, pepperoni and salt.

In a separate mixing bowl, stir together the tomato paste and egg.

Add egg and tomato paste mix to dry ingredients and stir.

Using a rubber spatula, pour / scoop the waffle batter into the center of the iron. Lightly moisten your fingers to prevent sticking and press the waffle dough evenly to the edges of the waffle wells.

Close the iron with a light press to the top to make sure all ingredients are spread evenly. Be careful not to press the hot parts of your iron. **Bake briefly for around 3 minutes on 100% heat.**

Lift the lid to check for desired color. Remove by lifting an edge with a fork at the tip of a waffle ridge. Slide a spatula underneath and towards the center. Lift / slide to a cutting board or cooling rack.

Allow to cool briefly and enjoy!

Tips: **Make it pesto:** Swap out the tomato paste for pesto sauce for a sweet twist.

Mix in the ranch?! Swap out 1 Tbsp of tomato paste for 1 Tbsp Ranch dressing.

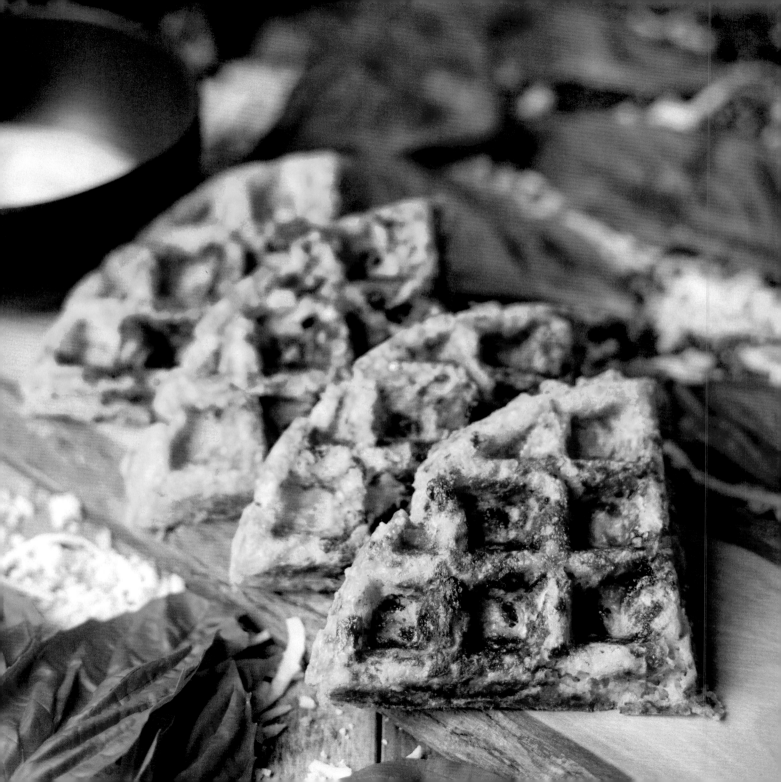

CAJUN PESTO

An old favorite flavor mix of mine with a new low carb twist. Sweet pesto flavor up front, with a nice spicy afterthought all wrapped into a cheesy crunch. The smell alone from the moment it hits the iron is amazingly mouth watering. Check out the tips at the bottom of the page for a simple Cajun spice recipe.

Prep: 5 Minutes	Cook: 4 Minutes	Total: 9 Minutes

Almond Flour	1/4 Cup
Raw Riced Cauliflower	1/4 Cup
Shredded Parmesan Cheese	1/4 Cup
Shredded Mozzarella Cheese	1/2 Cup
Cajun Seasoning	1 1/2 Tsp
Pesto	2 Tbsp
Large Egg(s)	1

Plug in a clean waffle iron and set the temperature to **100% heat.**

In a medium sized mixing bowl, stir together the almond flour, raw riced cauliflower, cheese and Cajun seasoning.

In the same mixing bowl, stir in the pesto and egg

Using a rubber spatula, pour / scoop the waffle batter into the center of the iron. Lightly moisten your fingers to prevent sticking and press the waffle dough evenly to the edges of the waffle wells.

Close the iron with a light press to the top to make sure all ingredients are spread evenly. Be careful not to press the hot parts of the iron. **Bake briefly for around 4 minutes on 100% heat.**

Lift the lid to check for desired color. Remove by lifting an edge with a fork at the tip of a waffle ridge. Slide a spatula underneath and towards the center. Lift / slide to a cutting board or cooling rack.

Allow to cool briefly and enjoy!

Tips: **Make your own Cajun Spice:**
Mix in a separate bowl
Store extra for later recipes

1 Tbsp Paprika
1 Tbsp Garlic powder
1 Tbsp Cayenne pepper

1 Tbsp White pepper
1 Tbsp Onion powder
1 Tbsp Black pepper

CAJUN PESTO
ROAST BEEF

Slice up some roast beef.
Cut some tomato.
Tear off some lettuce.
Stack between two Cajun Pesto waffles (hot or cold).
No mayo needed.
You've got yourself a sandwich.

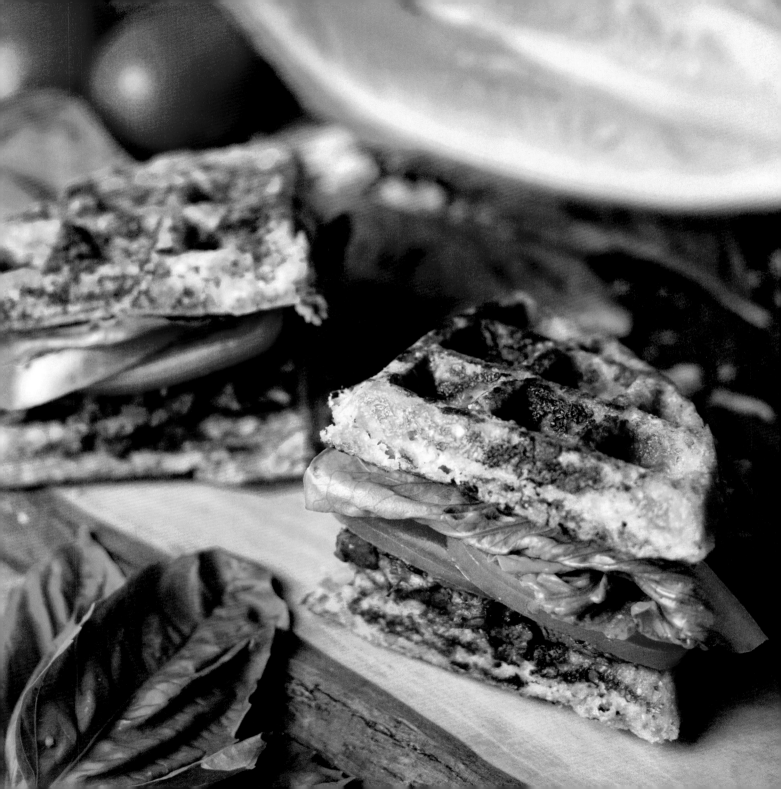

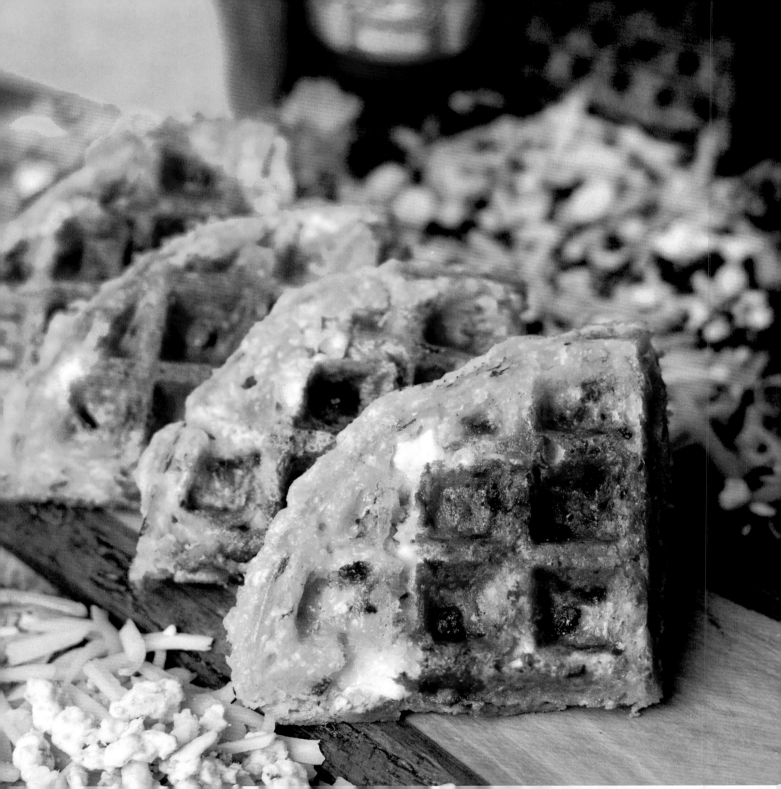

CHEDDAR BUFFALO BLUE

Before I wrote this recipe I wasn't a huge fan of buffalo sauce. This waffle completely changed that opinion. The creamy cooling effect that the melted blue cheese adds into the sweet spice of the buffalo sauce with a nice bit of bite from the cheddar all wrapped into a delicious crunch hits it out of the park.

Prep: 5 Minutes	Cook: 4 Minutes	Total: 9 Minutes

Almond Flour	1/4 Cup
Raw Riced Cauliflower	1/4 Cup
Shredded Mozzarella Cheese	1/4 Cup
Shredded Mild Cheddar Cheese	1/2 Cup
Buffalo Sauce	2 Tbsp
Large Egg(s)	1
Crumbled Blue Cheese	1/4 Cup

Plug in a clean waffle iron and set the temperature to **100% heat.**

In a medium sized mixing bowl, stir together the almond flour, raw riced cauliflower and cheese. (Keep the blue cheese separate for later.)

In the same mixing bowl, stir in the buffalo sauce and egg.

Using a rubber spatula, pour / scoop the waffle batter into the center of the iron.

Spread the ingredients to about ¼ inch away from the edges of the waffle wells. Place the ¼ cup of crumbled blue cheese on top of the batter and spread out evenly. Pressing the batter out the rest of the way to the edges of the waffle wells.

Close the iron with a light press to the top to make sure all ingredients are spread evenly. Be careful not to press the hot parts of your iron. **Bake briefly for around 4 minutes on 100% heat.**

Lift the lid to check for desired color. Remove by lifting an edge with a fork at the tip of a waffle ridge. Slide a spatula underneath and towards the center. Lift / slide to a cutting board or cooling rack.

Allow to cool briefly and enjoy!

Tips: **Does it have to go on top?** Yes, the blue cheese gets too melty to be mixed directly in.

Not a fan of blue cheese? Ditch it and add an extra 1/4 cup of mozzarella for a Cheddar Buffalo waffle.

CHEDDAR BUFFALO BLUE SHREDDED CHICKEN

Slice up some chicken thighs (or breast).
Cut some tomato slices.
Tear off some lettuce.
Stack between two Cheddar Buffalo Blue waffles (hot or cold).
No mayo needed.
You've got yourself a sandwich.

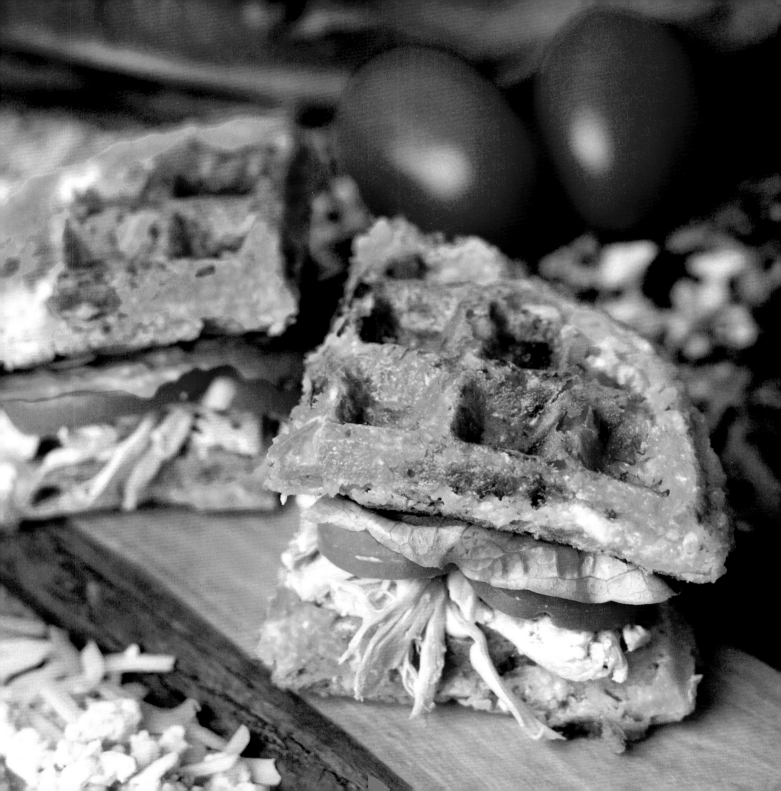

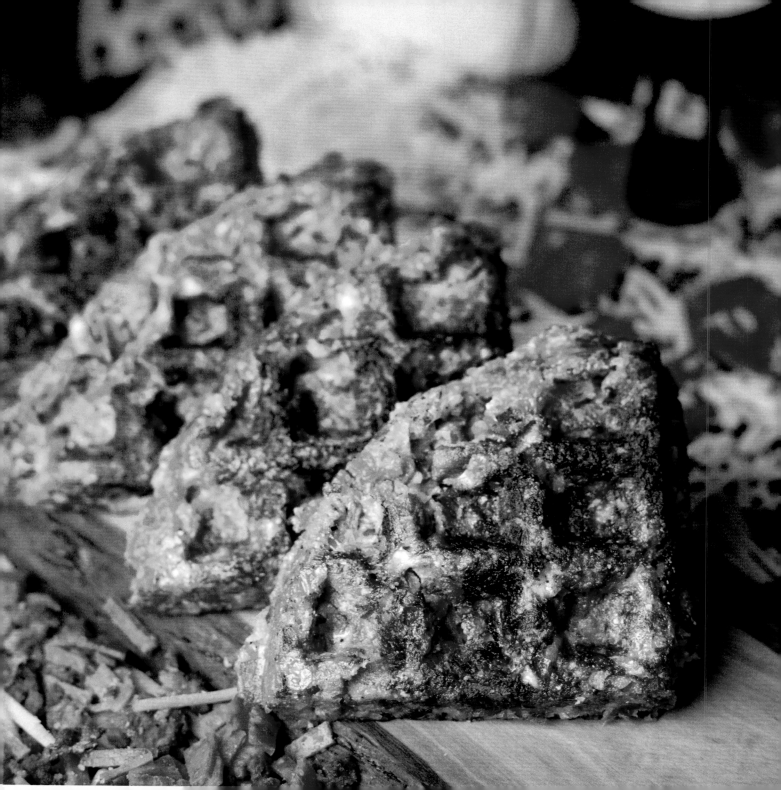

THREE MEAT PIZZA

Need some meat? Meet the Three Meat Pizza waffle.
For those times you want meat and you want pizza, but you don't want the bread.

Prep: 10 Minutes	Cook: 3 Minutes	Total: 13 Minutes

Almond Flour	1/4 Cup
Raw Riced Cauliflower	3 Tbsp
Shredded Mozzarella Cheese	1/4 Cup
Shredded Parmesan Cheese	1/2 Cup
Crumbled Bacon	1/4 Cup
Minced Italian Sausage (Cooked / Crumbled)	1/4 Cup
Minced Pepperoni	1/4 Cup
Tomato Paste	2 Tbsp
Large Egg(s)	1

Plug in a clean waffle iron and set the temperature to **100% heat.**

In a medium sized mixing bowl, stir together the almond flour, raw riced cauliflower, cheese, bacon, sausage and pepperoni.

In a separate mixing bowl, stir together the tomato paste and egg.

Add egg and tomato paste mix to dry ingredients and stir.

Using a rubber spatula, pour / scoop the waffle batter into the center of the iron. Lightly moisten your fingers to prevent sticking and press the waffle dough evenly to the edges of the waffle wells.

Close the iron with a light press to the top to make sure all ingredients are spread evenly. Be careful not to press the hot parts of the iron. **Bake briefly for around 3 minutes on 100% heat.**

Lift the lid to check for desired color. Remove by lifting an edge with a fork at the tip of a waffle ridge. Slide a spatula underneath and towards the center. Lift / slide to a cutting board or cooling rack.

Allow to cool briefly and enjoy!

Tips: **Don't want to fry some bacon?** Real bacon bits work just as great!

Mince it up: Make sure all your meats are well minced into a small size for a better fit.

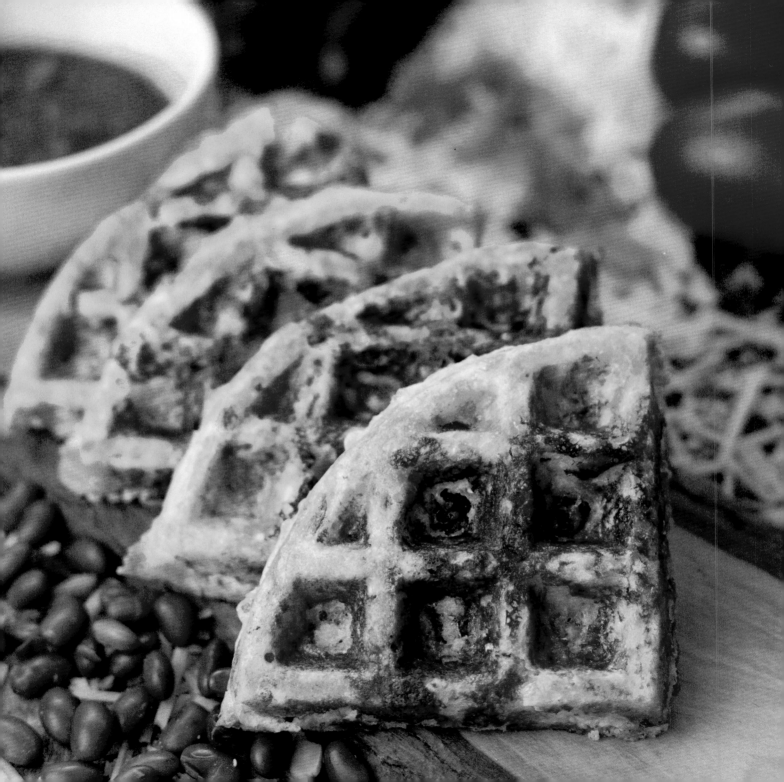

CRUNCHY ENCHILADA

The key to this recipe are the Organic Black Soy Beans from Eden foods. Spice, crunch and a fantastic hint of bean flavor, this waffle is a very different take on a dish it's almost nothing like. Trust me though, it's delicious.

Prep: 5 Minutes	Cook: 3 Minutes	Total: 8 Minutes

Almond Flour	1/4 Cup
Raw Riced Cauliflower	2 Tbsp
Shredded Parmesan Cheese	1/4 Cup
Shredded Mozzarella Cheese	1/2 Cup
Black Soy Beans (Drained/Rinsed)	1/4 Cup
Red Salsa	2 Tbsp
Canned Diced Green Chillies	1 Tbsp
Large Egg(s)	1

Plug in a clean waffle iron and set the temperature to **100% heat.**

In a medium sized mixing bowl, stir together the almond flour, raw riced cauliflower, cheese and black soy beans.

In the same mixing bowl, stir in the salsa, diced green chilies and egg.

Using a rubber spatula, pour / scoop the waffle batter into the center of the iron. Lightly moisten your fingers to prevent sticking and press the waffle dough evenly to the edges of the waffle wells.

Close the iron with a light press to the top to make sure all ingredients are spread evenly. Be careful not to press the hot parts of the iron. **Bake briefly for around 3 minutes on 100% heat.**

Lift the lid to check for desired color. Remove by lifting an edge with a fork at the tip of a waffle ridge. Slide a spatula underneath and towards the center. Lift / slide to a cutting board or cooling rack.

Allow to cool briefly and enjoy!

 Tips:

Looking for more crunch? Let it go a minute longer.

Can't find the beans? Check their website, edenfoods.com/store

CRUNCHY ENCHILADA
AVOCADO ROAST BEEF

Slice up some roast beef.
Cut some avocado slices.
Tear off some lettuce.
Stack between two Crunchy Enchilada waffles (hot or cold).
You've got yourself a sandwich.

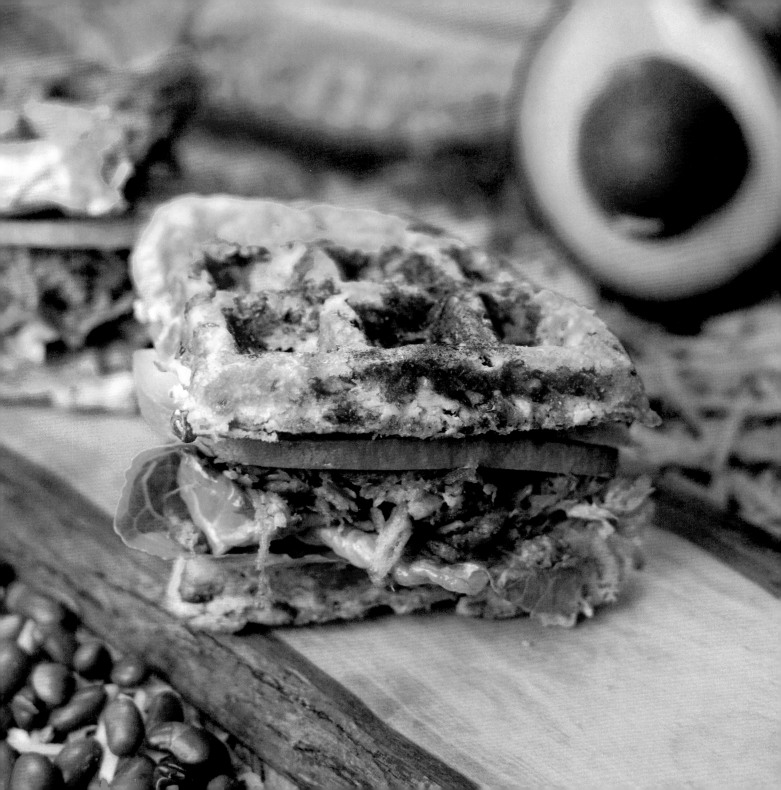

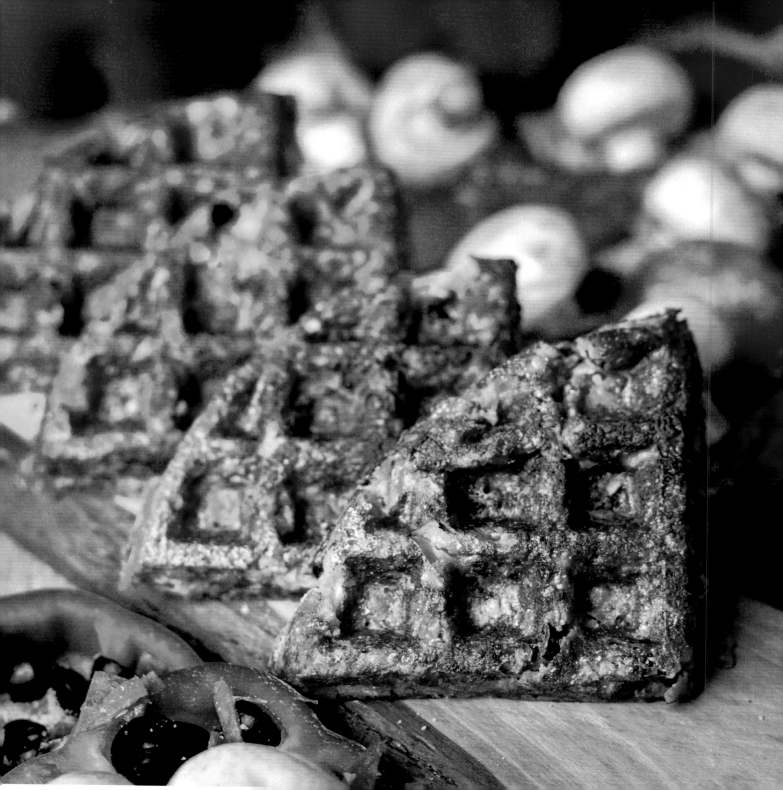

Supreme Pizza

So much pizza flavor packed into one waffle. Getting everything packed into the waffle iron took quite of bit of trial and error, but it was well worth the challenge.

Prep: 15 Minutes	Cook: 4 Minutes	Total: 19 Minutes

Almond Flour	1/4 Cup
Shredded Parmesan Cheese	1/2 Cup
Raw Riced Cauliflower	2 Tbsp
Minced Green Bell Peppers	2 Tbsp
Minced Mushrooms	2 Tbsp
Minced Olives	2 Tbsp
Minced Pepperoni	2 Tbsp
Minced ItalianSausage (Cooked / Crumbled)	2 Tbsp
Tomato Paste	2 Tbsp
Large Egg(s)	1

Plug in a clean waffle iron and set the temperature to **100% heat.**

In a medium sized mixing bowl, stir together the almond flour, cheese, raw riced cauliflower, green bell pepper, mushrooms, olives, pepperoni and sausage

In a separate mixing bowl, stir together the tomato paste and egg.

Add egg and tomato paste mix to dry ingredients and stir.

Using a rubber spatula, pour / scoop the waffle batter into the center of the iron. Lightly moisten your fingers to prevent sticking and press the waffle dough evenly to the edges of the waffle wells.

Close the iron with a light press to the top to make sure all ingredients are spread evenly and that the iron closes all the way. Be careful not to press the hot parts of the iron. **Bake briefly for around 4 minutes on 100% heat.**

Lift the lid to check for desired color. Remove by lifting an edge with a fork at the tip of a waffle ridge. Slide a spatula underneath and towards the center. Lift / slide to a cutting board or cooling rack.

Allow to cool briefly and enjoy!

Tips: **If cold pizza's your thing:** Like normal pizza, this waffle is also great as a leftover.

Mince it up: Make sure all your minced ingredients are nice and small for a better fit.

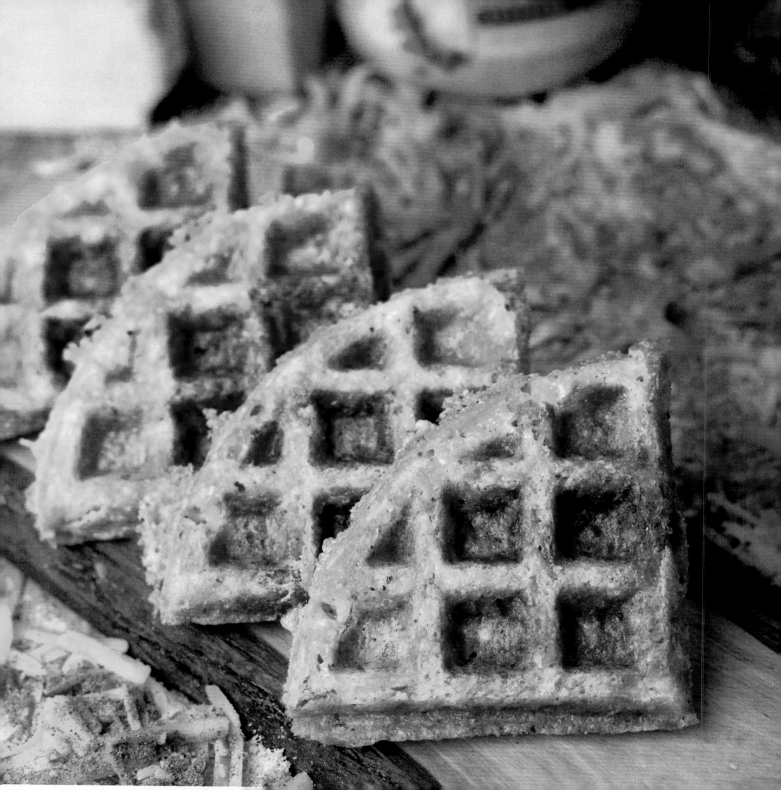

CAJUN CHEDDAR RANCH

A bit of spice, a bit of bite and a bit of cool.
The Cajun Cheddar Ranch waffle sends your senses through a rollercoaster of flavor.
Check the tips below to make your own Cajun spice.

Prep: 5 Minutes	Cook: 3 Minutes	Total: 8 Minutes

Almond Flour	1/4 Cup
Raw Riced Cauliflower	1/4 Cup
Shredded Parmesan Cheese	1/4 Cup
Shredded Mild Cheddar Cheese	1/2 Cup
Ranch	2 Tbsp
Cajun Seasoning	1 1/2 Tsp
Large Egg(s)	1

Plug in a clean waffle iron and set the temperature to **100% heat.**

In a medium sized mixing bowl, stir together the almond flour, raw riced cauliflower, cheese, and Cajun seasoning.

In the same mixing bowl, stir in the ranch dressing and egg.

Using a rubber spatula, pour / scoop the waffle batter into the center of the iron. Lightly moisten your fingers to prevent sticking and press the waffle dough evenly to the edges of the waffle wells.

Close the iron with a light press to the top to make sure all ingredients are spread evenly. Be careful not to press the hot parts of the iron. **Bake briefly for around 3 minutes on 100% heat.**

Lift the lid to check for desired color. Remove by lifting an edge with a fork at the tip of a waffle ridge. Slide a spatula underneath and towards the center. Lift / slide to a cutting board or cooling rack.

Allow to cool briefly and enjoy!

 Tips: **Make your own Cajun Spice:**

Mix in a separate bowl
Store extra for later recipes

1 Tbsp Paprika
1 Tbsp Garlic powder
1 Tbsp Cayenne pepper

1 Tbsp White pepper
1 Tbsp Onion powder
1 Tbsp Black pepper

CAJUN CHEDDAR RANCH BACON LETTUCE... TUNA?

Mix up a can of Tuna.
Fry a bit of bacon.
Tear off some lettuce.
Stack between two Cajun Cheddar Ranch waffles (hot or cold).
You've got yourself a sandwich.

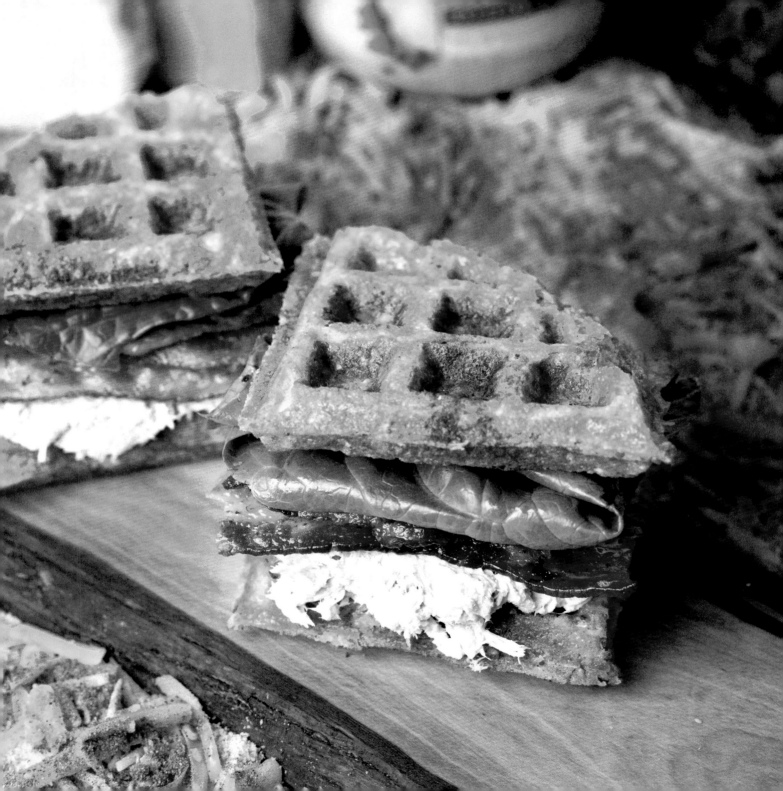

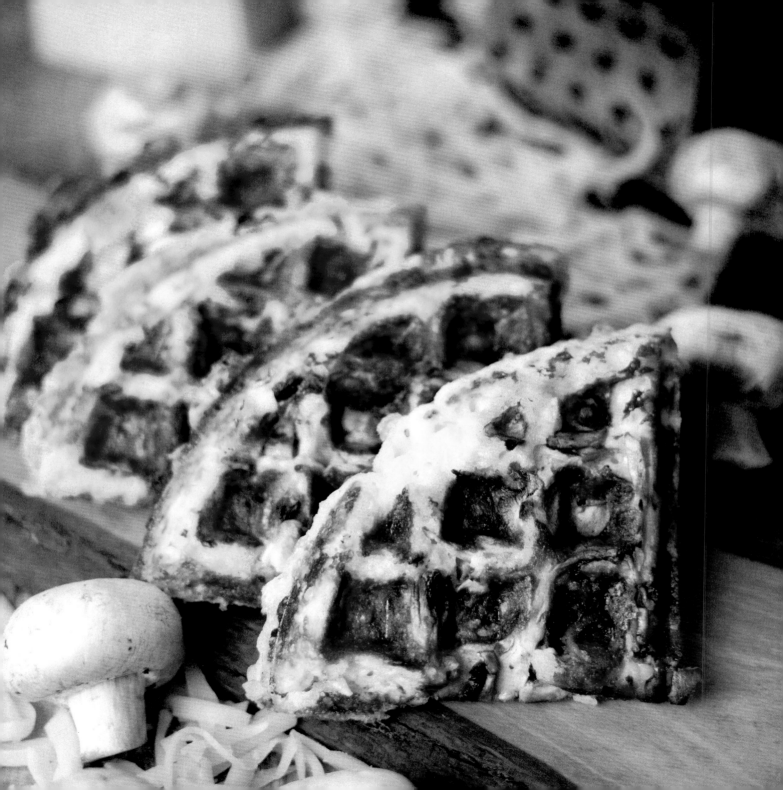

MUSHROOM SWISS

Something about the soft texture of the mushrooms mixed with the smooth creaminess of a delicious swiss cheese just makes this waffle the perfect combo of flavors. Simple in its creation but complex in flavor. This waffle is an instant hit with many.

Prep: 5 Minutes	Cook: 4 Minutes	Total: 9 Minutes

Almond Flour	1/4 Cup
Shredded Mozzarella Cheese	1/2 Cup
Shredded Swiss Cheese	1/2 Cup
Heavy Whipping Cream	1 Tbsp
Large Egg(s)	1
Diced Mushrooms	1/2 Cup

Plug in a clean waffle iron and set the temperature to **100% heat.**

In a medium sized mixing bowl, stir together the almond flour and cheese.
(save the mushrooms for a later step)

In the same mixing bowl, stir in the heavy whipping cream and egg.

Using a rubber spatula, pour / scoop the waffle batter into the center of the iron.

Spread the ingredients to about ½ inch away from the edges of the waffle wells. Place your ½ cup of diced mushrooms on top of the batter and spread out evenly. Lightly moisten your fingers to prevent sticking and press the waffle dough evenly to the edges of the waffle wells.

Close the iron with a light press to the top to make sure all ingredients are spread evenly. Be careful not to press the hot parts of the iron. **Bake briefly for around 4 minutes on 100% heat.**

Lift the lid to check for desired color. Remove by lifting an edge with a fork at the tip of a waffle ridge. Slide a spatula underneath and towards the center. Lift / slide to a cutting board or cooling rack.

Allow to cool briefly and enjoy!

 Tips: **Spice it up:** Add 1 Tsp of cajun spice for an extra twist of flavor.

Freeze Them! Store any leftovers in the freezer! Re-heat in an iron or toaster oven!

MUSHROOM SWISS BURGER

Fry up a burger patty.
Slice up a tomato.
Tear off some lettuce.
Shred some swiss cheese.
Stack between two Mushroom Swiss waffles (hot or cold).
You've got yourself a burger.

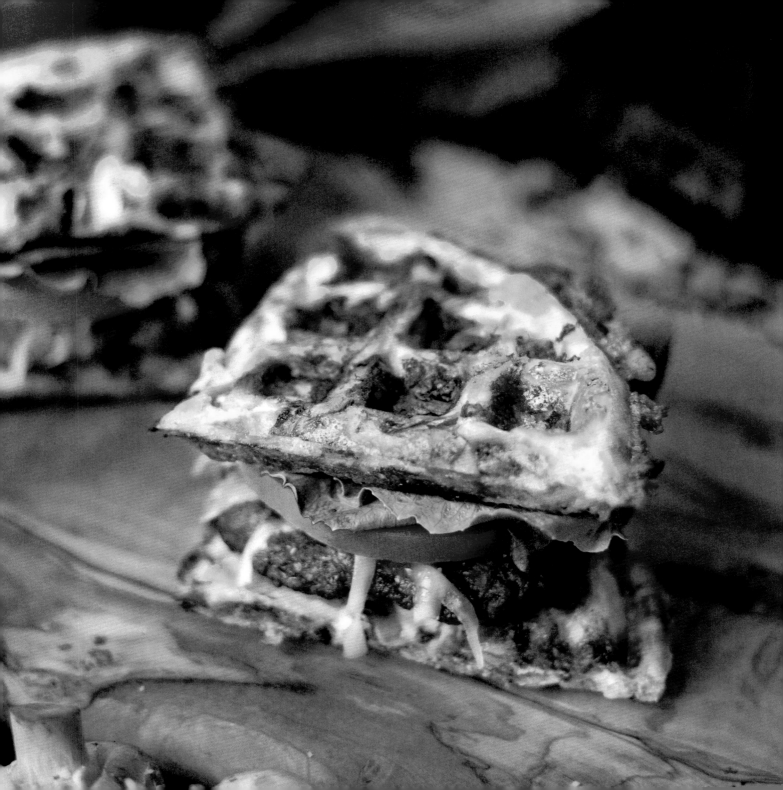

MUSHROOM SWISS PEPPERONI PIZZA

Grate some Mozzarellla cheese.
Set your waffle iron to 25% heat.
Place half of a Mushroom Swiss Waffle in the front half of Your Iron.
Place grated cheese on top of those waffles.
Layer pepperoni slices on the cheese.
Stack the other half of the waffle on top.
Close your iron lightly and allow to cook till the cheese is melted.
You've got yourself a pizza sandwich.

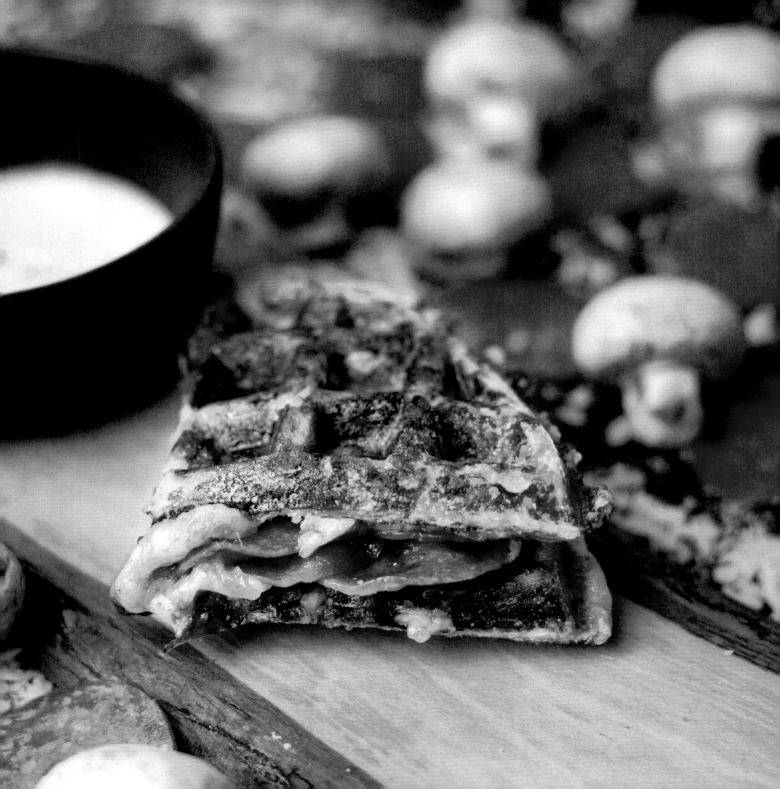

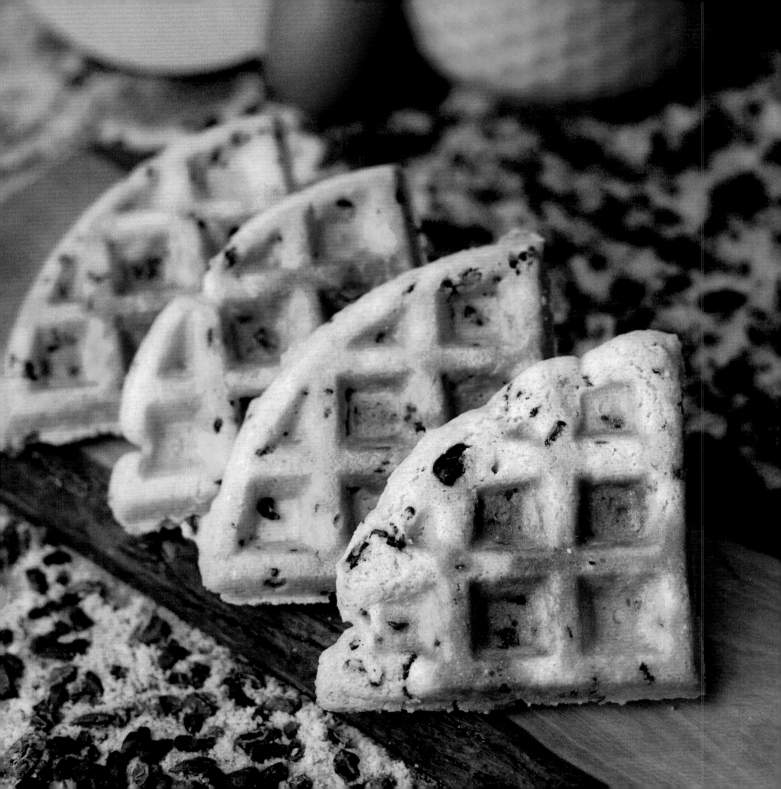

Cocoa Nib Cookie

The best low carb and gluten free "Chocolate chip" cookie I've ever made.
Better when cooled, even better when frozen.

Prep: 5 Minutes	Cook: 5 Minutes	Total: 10 Minutes

Almond Flour	3/4 Cup
Cocoa Nibs	3 Tbsp
Pyure Stevia Blend	3 Tbsp
Melted Butter	1 1/2 Tbsp
Heavy Whipping Cream	1 Tbsp
Large Egg(s)	1

Plug in your clean waffle iron and set your temperature to **50% heat.**

In a medium sized mixing bowl, stir together the almond flour, stevia and cocoa nibs.

In a separate mixing bowl, stir together the melted butter, heavy whipping cream and egg.

Add liquids mix to dry ingredients and stir.

Using a rubber spatula, pour / scoop the waffle batter into the center of the iron. Lightly moisten your fingers to prevent sticking and press the waffle dough evenly to the edges of the waffle wells.

Close the iron with a light press to the top to make sure all ingredients are spread evenly. Be careful not to press the hot parts of the iron. **Bake briefly for around 5 minutes on 50% heat.**

Lift the lid to check for desired color. Unplug the iron and allow the it to cool for around 10 minutes before using your rubber spatula to slice into individual triangles. Remove one at a time by sliding your spatula under and lifting each one individually.

Enjoy!

Tips:

Cut it again: Slice the waffle quarters into eighths for a better serving size.

Keep it cool: Store them in the freezer for a longer shelf life... If the'yre not eaten right away.

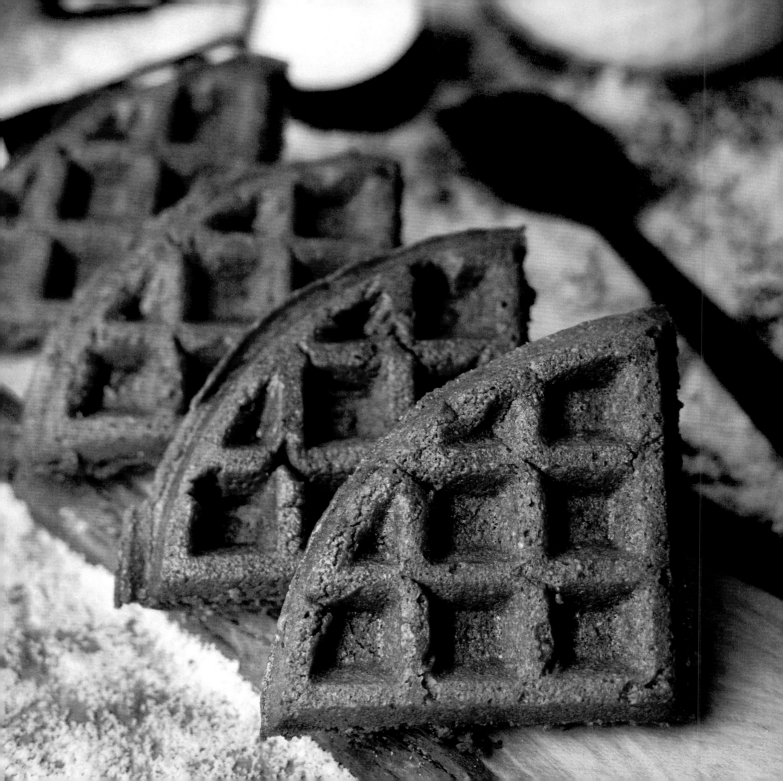

THREE STAGE FUDGE BROWNIE

On first removal the top half of the brownie maintains a light crunch while the bottom and center are still warm and gooey. As the waffle cools, both sides develop a crunch with a moist center. Stored for later, the brownie takes on a completely different and delicious texture.

Prep: 5 Minutes	Cook: 8 Minutes	Total: 13 Minutes

Almond Flour	1 Cup
Pyure Stevia Blend	1/3 Cup
Unsweetened Cocoa Powder	2 Tbsp
Salt	1/4 Tsp
Gelatin	1 Packet
Melted Butter	3 1/2 Tbsp
Heavy Whipping Cream	2 Tbsp
Large Egg(s)	1

Plug in a clean waffle iron and set the temperature to **25% heat.**

In a medium sized mixing bowl, stir together

the almond flour, stevia, unsweetened cocoa powder, salt and gelatin.

In a separate mixing bowl, stir together the melted butter, heavy whipping cream and egg.

Add liquids mix to dry ingredients and stir.

Using a rubber spatula, pour / scoop the waffle batter into the center of the iron. Lightly moisten your fingers to prevent sticking and press the waffle dough evenly to the edges of the waffle wells.

Close the iron with a light press to the top to make sure all ingredients are spread evenly. Be careful not to press the hot parts of the iron. **Bake briefly for around 8 minutes on 25% heat.**

Lift the lid to check for desired color. Unplug the iron and allow it to cool for around 10 minutes. Use a rubber spatula to cut the waffle into individual triangles along the waffle ridges. Remove one at a time by lifting the waffle along the outer waffle wells, sliding a spatula under and lifting each one individually to a cutting board or cooling rack.

Enjoy!

 Tips: **Buying in bulk?** 1 packet of gelatin comes out to roughly 0.25 oz.

Cut it again: Slice the waffle quarters into eighths for a better serving size.

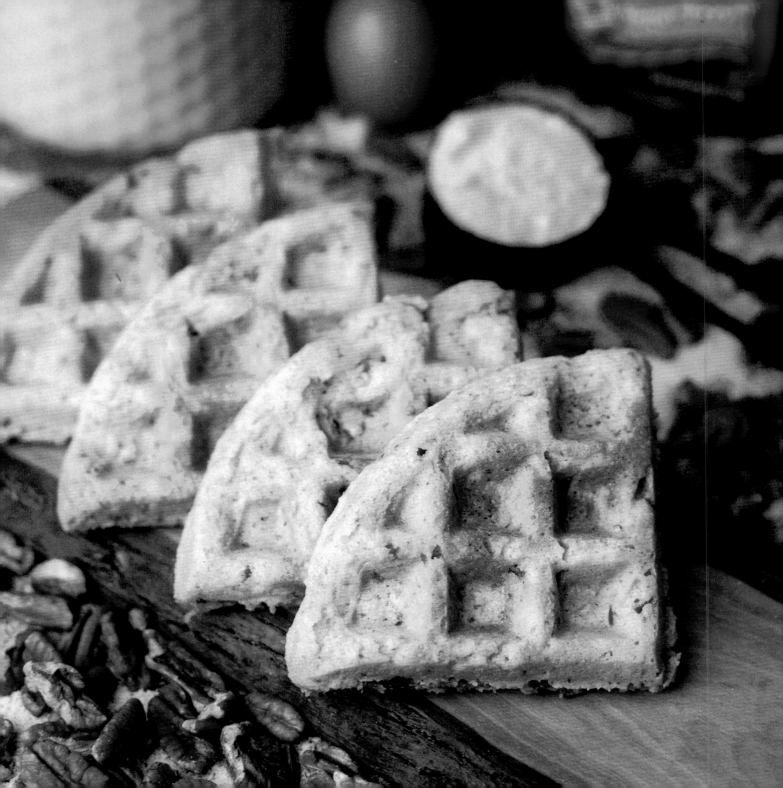

Maple Pecan Cookie

Sweet maple flavor mixed with a buttery pecan crunch all into one amazingly low carb waffle cookie.

Prep: 5 Minutes	Cook: 5 Minutes	Total: 10 Minutes

Almond Flour	3/4 Cup
Pyure Stevia Blend	3 Tbsp
Crushed Pecans	1/4 Cup
Melted Butter	2 Tbsp
Sugar Free Maple Syrup	2 Tbsp
Large Egg(s)	1

Plug in your clean waffle iron and set your temperature to **50% heat.**

In a medium sized mixing bowl, stir together the almond flour, stevia, and crushed pecans.

In a separate mixing bowl, stir together the melted butter, sugar free maple syrup and egg.

Add liquids mix to dry ingredients and stir.

Using a rubber spatula, pour / scoop the waffle batter into the center of the iron. Lightly moisten your fingers to prevent sticking and press the waffle dough evenly to the edges of the waffle wells.

Close your iron with a light press to the top to make sure all ingredients are spread evenly. Be careful not to press the hot parts of the iron. **Bake briefly for around 5 minutes on 50% heat.**

Lift the lid to check for desired color. Unplug the iron and allow it to cool for around 10 minutes. Use a rubber spatula to cut the waffle into individual triangles along the waffle ridges. Remove one at a time by lifting the waffle along the outer waffle wells, sliding a spatula under and lifting each one individually to a cutting board or cooling rack.

Enjoy!

Tips:

Baking Pecans? Pre-roasted or ones ment for baking, both will work here.

Cut it again: Slice the waffle quarters into eighths for a better serving size.

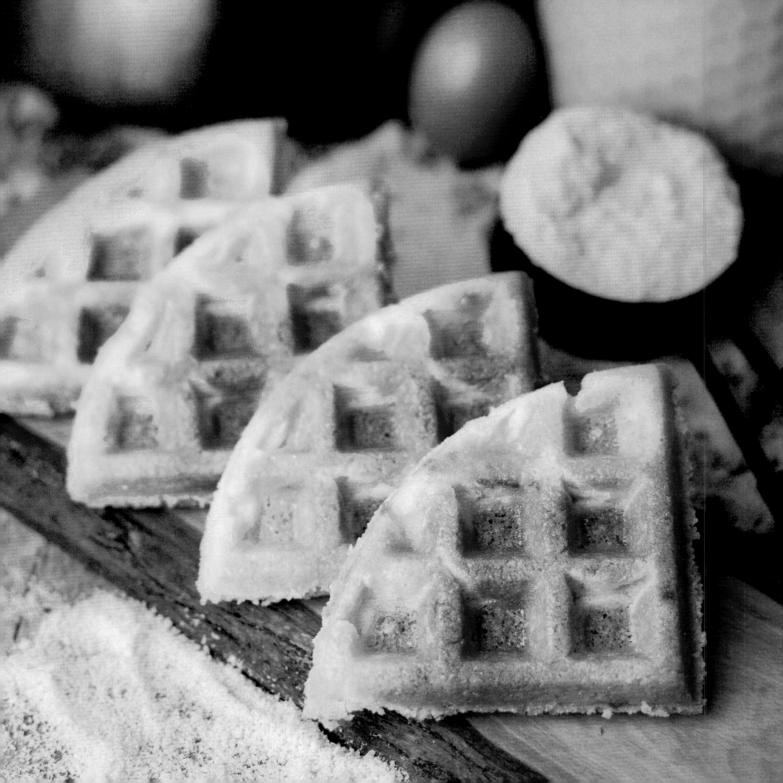

CAKE

Enjoyed plain with a cup of coffee or coated with a cream cheese frosting, the cake waffle is just the right sweet for almost any time of the day.

Prep: 5 Minutes	Cook: 10 Minutes	Total: 15 Minutes

Almond Flour	1 Cup
Pyure Stevia Blend	1/4 Cup
Gelatin	1 Packet
Melted Butter	3 Tbsp
Heavy Whipping Cream	1 Tbsp
Vanilla	1/4 Tsp
Large Egg(s)	1

Plug in a clean waffle iron and set the temperature to **25% heat.**

In a medium sized mixing bowl, stir together the almond flour, stevia and gelatin.

In a separate mixing bowl, stir together the melted butter, heavy whipping cream, vanilla and egg.

Add liquids mix to dry ingredients and stir.

Using a rubber spatula, pour / scoop the waffle batter into the center of the iron. Lightly moisten your fingers to prevent sticking and press the waffle dough evenly to the edges of the waffle wells.

Close your iron with a light press to the top to make sure all ingredients are spread evenly. Be careful not to press the hot parts of the iron. **Bake briefly for around 10 minutes on 25% heat.**

Lift the lid to check for desired color. Unplug the iron and allow it to cool for around 10 minutes. Use a rubber spatula to cut the waffle into individual triangles along the waffle ridges. Remove one at a time by lifting the waffle along the outer waffle wells, sliding a spatula under and lifting each one individually to a cutting board or cooling rack.

Enjoy!

Tips: **Buying in bulk?** 1 packet of gelatin comes out to roughly 0.25 oz.

Cut it again: Slice the waffle quarters into eighths for a better serving size.

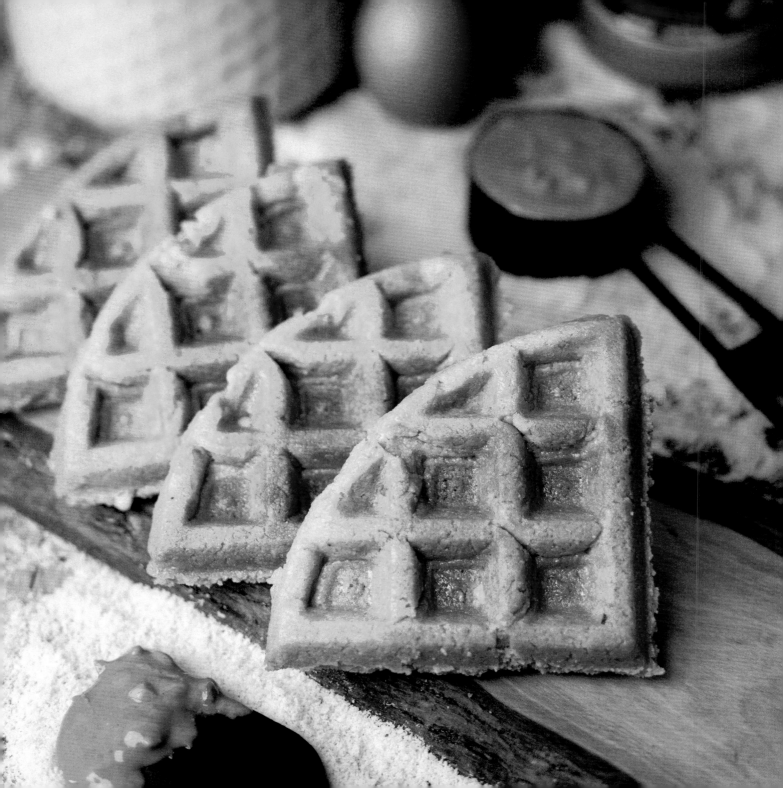

PEANUT BUTTER COOKIE

How could I make cookies in a waffle iron and not find a way to make a low carb peanut butter version? These surely hit that classic flavor and crunch without all the carbs.

Prep: 5 Minutes	Cook: 10 Minutes	Total: 15 Minutes

Almond Flour	2/3 Cup
Pyure Stevia Blend	1/4 Cup
Natural Peanut Butter	1/3 Cup
Melted Butter	2 Tbsp
Heavy Whipping Cream	1 Tbsp
Vanilla	1/4 Tsp
Large Egg(s)	1

Plug in a clean waffle iron and set the temperature to **50% heat.**

In a medium sized mixing bowl, stir together the almond flour, stevia, and salt.

In a separate mixing bowl, stir together the natural peanut butter, melted butter, vanilla and egg.

Add liquids mix to dry ingredients and stir.

Using a rubber spatula, pour / scoop the waffle batter into the center of the iron. Lightly moisten your fingers to prevent sticking and press the waffle dough evenly to the edges of the waffle wells.

Close the iron with a light press to the top to make sure all ingredients are spread evenly. Be careful not to press the hot parts of the iron. **Bake briefly for around 10 minutes on 50% heat.**

Lift the lid to check for desired color. Unplug the iron and allow it to cool for around 10 minutes. Use a rubber spatula to cut the waffle into individual triangles along the waffle ridges. Remove one at a time by lifting the waffle along the outer waffle wells, sliding a spatula under and lifting each one individually to a cutting board or cooling rack.

Enjoy!

Tips:

Keep it cool: Store them in the refrigerator for a longer shelf life.

Cut it again: Slice the waffle quarters into eighths for a better serving size.

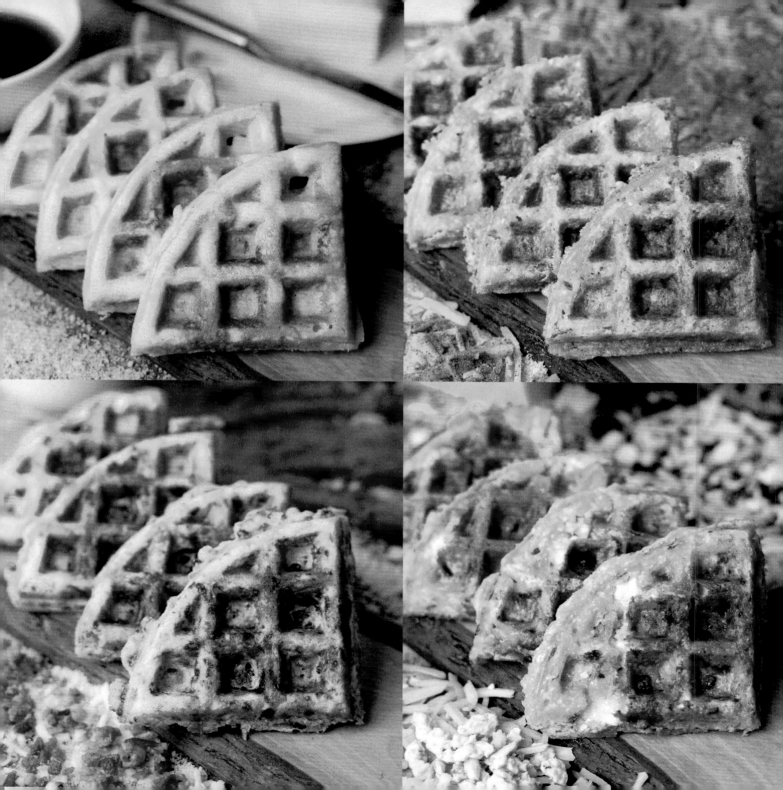

NUTRITIONAL ESTIMATIONS

Why, "Nutritional Estimations"? Because these numbers are based off the ingredients that I purchased and used for the recipes. Your ingredients may vary. As with any diet, it's always useful to still remain mindful of the products you're purchasing and using. These estimations are to give a general idea.

Almond Flour Classic

4 servings per waffle	Per Serving	Whole Waffle
Servings	1	4
Calories	117	470
Fat	9.5 g	38g
Protein	1.8 g	7 g
NET Carbs	2 g	8 g

Blueberry Muffin

4 servings per waffle	Per Serving	Whole Waffle
Servings	1	4
Calories	166	664
Fat	12 g	48 g
Protein	4.3 g	17 g
NET Carbs	4.5 g	18 g

Cake

8 servings per waffle	Per Serving	Whole Waffle
Servings	1	8
Calories	73	582
Fat	5.5 g	44 g
Protein	1 g	7 g
NET Carbs	1.5 g	12 g

Cajun Cheddar Ranch

4 servings per waffle	Per Serving	Whole Waffle
Servings	1	4
Calories	141	564
Fat	12 g	45 g
Protein	7.3 g	29 g
NET Carbs	2 g	8 g

Cajun Pesto

4 servings per waffle	Per Serving	Whole Waffle
Servings	1	4
Calories	113	452
Fat	10 g	41 g
Protein	8.3 g	33 g
NET Carbs	1.8 g	7 g

Cheddar Buffalo Blue

4 servings per waffle	Per Serving	Whole Waffle
Servings	1	4
Calories	102	410
Fat	6.8 g	27 g
Protein	6.8 g	27 g
NET Carbs	1.8 g	7 g

NET carbs = Total Carbs - Fiber

NUTRITIONAL ESTIMATIONS

Cocoa Nib Cookie

8 servings per waffle	Per Serving	Whole Waffle
Servings	1	8
Calories	67.8	543
Fat	4.8 g	38 g
Protein	1.3 g	10 g
NET Carbs	1.8 g	15 g

Crunchy Enchilada

4 servings per waffle	Per Serving	Whole Waffle
Servings	1	4
Calories	113	451
Fat	6.5 g	26 g
Protein	9 g	36 g
NET Carbs	2.5 g	10 g

French Toast

4 servings per waffle	Per Serving	Whole Waffle
Servings	1	4
Calories	81	324
Fat	4.3 g	17 g
Protein	6.3 g	25 g
NET Carbs	2 g	8 g

Maple Bacon

4 servings per waffle	Per Serving	Whole Waffle
Servings	1	4
Calories	117	466
Fat	7 g	28 g
Protein	4.3 g	17 g
NET Carbs	3 g	12 g

Maple On-The-Go

4 servings per waffle	Per Serving	Whole Waffle
Servings	1	4
Calories	105	420
Fat	5.8 g	23 g
Protein	6.3 g	25 g
NET Carbs	2.7 g	11 g

Maple Pecan Cookie

8 servings per waffle	Per Serving	Whole Waffle
Servings	1	8
Calories	76	605
Fat	6.2 g	49 g
Protein	1.3 g	10 g
NET Carbs	1.3 g	11 g

Mushroom Swiss

4 servings per waffle	Per Serving	Whole Waffle
Servings	1	4
Calories	129	515
Fat	9 g	36 g
Protein	8.3 g	33 g
NET Carbs	4 g	16 g

Peanut Butter Cookie

8 servings per waffle	Per Serving	Whole Waffle
Servings	1	8
Calories	111.7	893
Fat	9,3 g	74 g
Protein	3.5 g	28 g
NET Carbs	1.6 g	13 g

Nutritional Estimations

Pepper Jack Ranch

4 servings per waffle	Per Serving	Whole Waffle
Servings	1	4
Calories	155	618
Fat	12. g	51 g
Protein	7.8 g	31 g
NET Carbs	2.2 g	9 g

Pepperoni Pizza

4 servings per waffle	Per Serving	Whole Waffle
Servings	1	4
Calories	129	517
Fat	9 g	36 g
Protein	7.8 g	31 g
NET Carbs	3 g	12 g

Supreme Pizza

4 servings per waffle	Per Serving	Whole Waffle
Servings	1	4
Calories	111	443
Fat	6.8 g	27 g
Protein	7.8 g	31 g
NET Carbs	3,2 g	13 g

Three Cheese

4 servings per waffle	Per Serving	Whole Waffle
Servings	1	4
Calories	99	393
Fat	6.8 g	27 g
Protein	7.8 g	31 g
NET Carbs	2 g	8 g

Three Meat Pizza

4 servings per waffle	Per Serving	Whole Waffle
Servings	1	4
Calories	168	672
Fat	12 g	47 g
Protein	13 g	53 g
NET Carbs	2 g	8 g

Three Stage Fudge Brownie

8 servings per waffle	Per Serving	Whole Waffle
Servings	1	8
Calories	96	765
Fat	7 g	55 g
Protein	1.2 g	9 g
NET Carbs	2 g	16 g

NET carbs = Total Carbs - Fiber

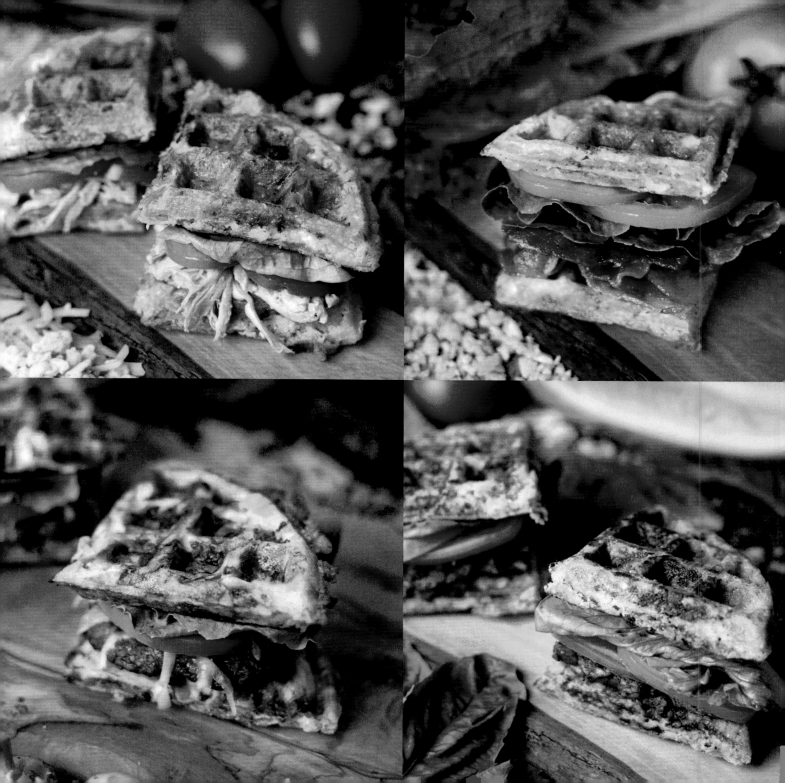

INDEX

Thanks For Reading!

I hope you've enjoyed these recipes
as much as I have.

Share your waffle creations on instagram with,

#WillOfTheWaffle

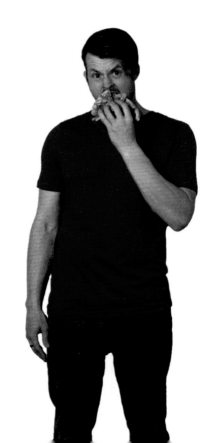

Made in the USA
San Bernardino, CA
11 August 2019